The Culinary Canvas of Bangladesh:
A Chef's Journey

By
Arfatul Islam,
MSc, Ulster University, UK

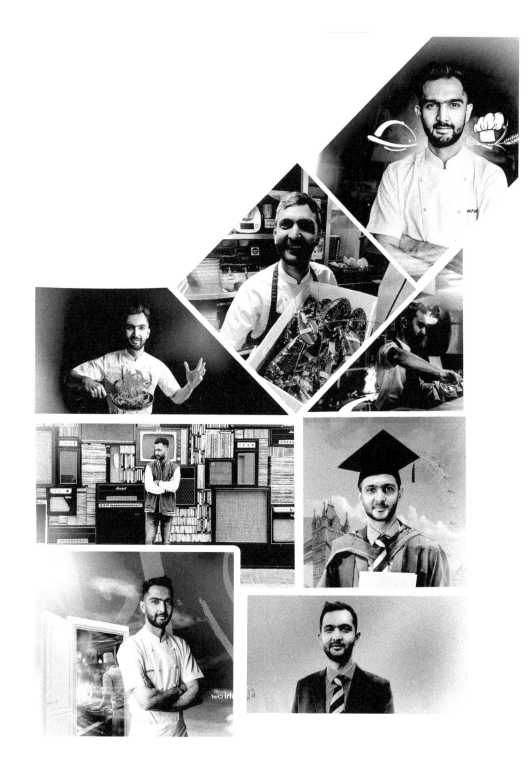

Introduction:

Greetings from the heart of Bangladesh, I am Arfatul Islam. I am a proud Bangladeshi, having studied in the prestigious Ulster University, UK, and crowned the topper for 2022. With a professional culinary certification at level 7, I am amongst the elite chefs in Bangladesh, Top chef in Bangladesh and UK .

This book encapsulates my personal journey through the rich and aromatic world of Bangladeshi cuisine. Drawing from a deep reservoir of culinary history and my own experiences, I have designed this book to illuminate the art of Bangladeshi cooking to novices and experts alike. It is my humble offering to my readers, my country, and the global culinary community.

"The Culinary Canvas of Bangladesh: A Chef's Journey" holds the distinction of being the first book to introduce Bangladeshi cuisine to a global audience. It is a comprehensive guide that goes beyond the realm of a traditional cookbook, offering a deep dive into the unique culinary traditions, culture, and history of Bangladesh.

This book does not incorporate any fictional elements, but rather focuses on providing accurate and authentic information about Bangladeshi cuisine. This authenticity sets the stage for future volumes that will continue to explore the evolving culinary landscape of Bangladesh.

We invite readers worldwide to purchase this book and delve into the exciting culinary world of Bangladesh. Not only will it expand your culinary repertoire, but it will also offer insights into a rich and diverse culture that has been largely unexplored on the global gastronomic scene.

By suggesting this book to others, you will be playing a crucial role in introducing and promoting Bangladeshi cuisine worldwide. This is an opportunity to be part of a movement that celebrates diversity, enriches culinary knowledge, and bridges cultural gaps through the universal language of food.

Arfatul Islam

Content

Chapter 1:
The Spice Trails

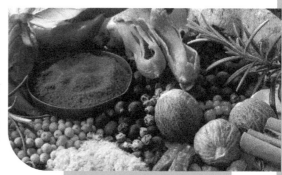

Welcome to the pulsating heart of Bangladesh: the bustling, vibrant spice markets. These are the places where culinary magic begins, and where you can taste the essence of Bangladesh in every grain.

Section 1.1: The Marketplaces

Spice markets in Bangladesh are the meeting points of tradition and commerce, the old and the new. Walking through the narrow, crowded lanes of these markets, you are greeted with a sensory overload. The aroma of spices fills the air, sacks full of vibrant colors catch your eye, and the chatter of shopkeepers haggling with customers rings in your ears.

Notable among these are Kawran Bazar in Dhaka and Chaktai Bazar in Chittagong. However, every city, every village has its own local market where you can find a vast variety of local and imported spices.

Section 1.2: The Spice Pantry

Bangladeshi cuisine is a masterful blend of different spices, each contributing its unique flavor, aroma, and health benefits. Some of the most frequently used spices include:

1. Cumin (Jeera) : Used in seed form or ground into a powder, cumin provides a warm and earthy flavor to dishes.

2. Turmeric (Halud) : Known for its bright yellow color and subtle earthy flavor, turmeric is a fundamental spice in Bangladeshi cooking and has numerous health benefits.

3. Coriander (Dhania) : Used as both fresh leaves and dried seeds, coriander provides a citrusy flavor and is often used in curries and biryanis.

4. Red Chili (Morich) : The heat in Bangladeshi cuisine often comes from red chili, used either fresh, dried, or in powdered form.

5. Panch Phoron : "Panch Phoron" is a traditional Bengali spice blend that translates to "five spices." This unique mixture is a staple in Bangladeshi cuisine and some parts of India, especially in the eastern regions. It's known for the depth of flavor it provides to a range of dishes.

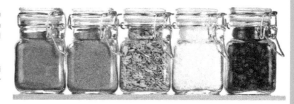

The five spices that make up Panch Phoron are:

1. **Fenugreek Seeds (Methi):** These seeds provide a somewhat bitter, burnt sugar taste.
2. **Nigella Seeds (Kalonji):** Nigella seeds have a slight onion-like flavor.
3. **Cumin Seeds (Jeera):** They lend a warm, earthy flavor to the mix.
4. **Black Mustard Seeds (Kalo Shorshe):** They contribute a strong, spicy kick.
5. **Fennel Seeds (Mouri):** Fennel seeds add a slightly sweet, anise-like flavor.

Unlike many spice mixes, Panch Phoron is used in its whole seed form rather than being ground up. The seeds are usually fried in oil or ghee (clarified butter), allowing them to release their flavors before other ingredients are added to the dish. This technique is called "tadka" or "tempering" and is a common method of cooking in the region.Panch Phoron is typically

Panch Phoron is typically used in dishes like lentils, vegetable stir-fries, fish, and even in pickles. Each of the five spices contributes a unique flavor profile, making Panch Phoron a multi-dimensional and versatile spice blend that enhances the flavor of a wide variety of dishes.

6. **Mustard (Shorshe):** Mustard seeds and mustard oil are fundamental ingredients, especially in fish dishes, providing a pungent and slightly bitter flavor.

Nutrition information
for each of the *spices* mentioned:

1. Cumin (Jeera):

Cumin is a staple spice in Bangladeshi cuisine. Its unique flavor is due to a compound called cuminaldehyde. Cumin also has potential health benefits, as it's rich in iron and has been linked to improved digestion and immune function.

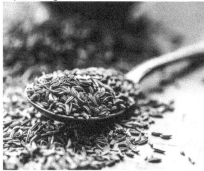

2. Turmeric (Halud):

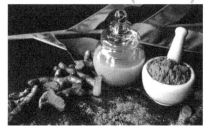

The active ingredient in turmeric is curcumin, which is known for its antiinflammatory and antioxidant properties. It's used in many dishes for its earthy flavor and vibrant yellow color.

- Nutritional Value:

Cumin seeds are low in calories and rich in essential nutrients.

- Macronutrients:

Cumin seeds are a good source of carbohydrates and dietary fiber.

- Micronutrients:

They contain various minerals like iron, manganese, magnesium, an calcium, aswell as vitamins like vitamin A, vitamin E, and vitamin C.

- Health Benefits:

Cumin is known for its potential digestive benefits, including aiding in digestion and reducing bloating and gas.

- Nutritional Value:

Turmeric is also low in calories but packed with essential nutrients.

- Macronutrients:

Turmeric contains carbohydrates, fiber, and a small amount of protein.

- Micronutrients:

It is a rich source of curcuminoids, especially curcumin, which has potent antioxidant and anti-inflammatory properties.

- Health Benefits:

Turmeric is renowned for its various health benefits, including its potential to reduce inflammation, support joint health, and promote overall well-being.

3. Coriander (Dhania):

Coriander seeds are used in Bangladeshi dishes for their warm, nutty flavor. They contain several compounds that act as antioxidants, promoting cellular health.

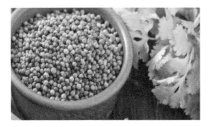

4. Red Chili (Morich):

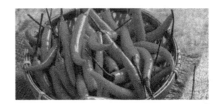

Chilies provide the heat in Bangladeshi dishes. The capsaicin in chili peppers is what gives them their spicy kick. Capsaicin also has health benefits, such as pain relief and cardiovascular health improvement.

- Nutritional Value:
Coriander leaves and seeds are low in calories and nutrient-dense.

- Macronutrients:
They provide carbohydrates, dietary fiber, and a small amount of protein.

- Micronutrients:
Coriander is rich in vitamins like vitamin A, vitamin C, vitamin K, and minerals like iron, calcium, and magnesium.

- Health Benefits:
Coriander may aid digestion and promote gut health due to its fiber content and potential antimicrobial properties

- Nutritional Value:
Turmeric is also low in calories but packed with essential nutrients.

- Macronutrients:
Turmeric contains carbohydrates, fiber, and a small amount of protein.

- Micronutrients:
It is a rich source of curcuminoids, especially curcumin, which has potent antioxidant and anti-inflammatory properties.

- Health Benefits:
Turmeric is renowned for its various health benefits, including its potential to reduce inflammation, support joint health, and promote overall well-being.

The science behind Panch Phoron involves the unique properties of its five spices: Fenugreek Seeds **(Methi):** They contain 4-hydroxyisoleucine, which can stimulate insulin production, and fiber for improved digestion

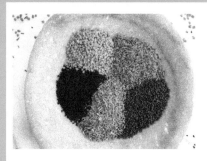

Nigella Seeds (Kalonji): Rich in thymoquinone, a potent antioxidant, anti-inflammatory, and anticancer compound.

Cumin Seeds (Jeera): A source of iron and antioxidants, they may help with weight loss and blood sugar regulation.

Black Mustard Seeds (Kalo Shorshe): They contain glucosinolates, studied for their anticancer properties, and are a source of anti-inflammatory selenium and magnesium.

Fennel Seeds (Mouri): High in fiber and containing anethole, a compound with potential anti-inflammatory and anticancer properties

These spices are typically heated in oil or ghee, enhancing their flavors and health benefits. However, they should complement, not replace, a balanced diet.

- Nutritional Value:
Panch Phoron is a combination of various seeds, providing a mix of nutrients from each component spice.

- Macronutrients:
It contains carbohydrates and dietary fiber.

- Micronutrients:
Panch Phoron includes fenugreek seeds, which may have potential health benefits related to blood sugar regulation.

- Health Benefits:
he individual spices in Panch Phoron contribute to its potential health benefits, which include supporting digestion and overall well-being.

6. Mustard (Shorshe):

These are often ground into a paste and used in Bengali fish dishes. They contain compounds called glucosinolates, which can transform into isothiocyanates, with potential anti-cancer properties.

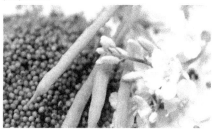

- Nutritional Value:
Mustard seeds and mustard oil are rich in essential nutrients.

- Macronutrients:
Mustard seeds contain carbohydrates, dietary fiber, and a small amount of protein.

- Micronutrients:
They are a good source of minerals like selenium, magnesium, and phosphorus, as well as vitamins like vitamin B6 and vitamin E.

- Health Benefits:
Mustard seeds and mustard oil have potential antioxidant and antimicrobial properties, and in moderation, they may contribute to a healthy diet.

Section 1.3: Spice Blends and Pastes

The magic of Bangladeshi cuisine lies in the unique combinations of these spices. Spice blends and pastes like bhorta (mashed preparations), paturi (marinated and steamed or grilled in banana leaves), and korma (braised dishes with yogurt, cream, and nut or seed paste) all use a complex medley of spices to create layered flavors.

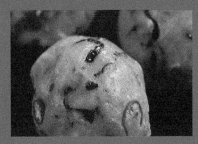

The Alchemy of Spices in Bangladeshi Cuisine

When you delve deep into Bangladeshi cuisine, it's evident that its heart lies in the meticulous use of spices. Beyond lending aromatic and intricate flavors, these spices play a pivotal role in maintaining a balanced diet, offering therapeutic and medicinal properties.

Bhorta
(Mashed Preparations)

Overview: Bhorta is a versatile preparation made by mashing boiled or roasted vegetables with spices, often including garlic, green chilli, and mustard oil.

Health Benefits:

1. Mustard Oil: A rich source of omega-3 fatty acids, it helps reduce heart disease risk.

2. Garlic: Known for its anti-inflammatory properties, it also aids in improving cardiovascular health.

3. Chilli: Contains capsaicin which boosts metabolism and promotes fat burning.

also known as "Chili Mash," is a spicy and flavorful Bangladeshi dish made from green chilies. It's a condiment that adds a fiery kick to your meals. Here's a simple recipe to make Chilli Bhorta:

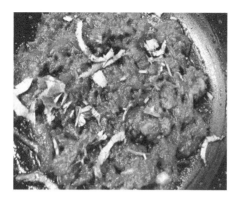

Chilli Bhorta

Ingredients:

Green chilies: 200 grams (adjust quantity based on your spice tolerance)
Onion: 1 small, finely chopped
Garlic: 3-4 cloves, minced
Mustard oil: 2-3 tablespoons
Salt: to taste
Lemon juice: From half a lemon

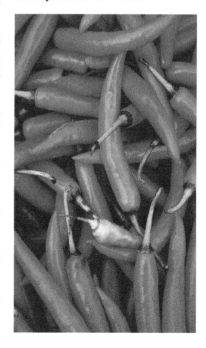

Instructions:

Prepare the Green Chilies:
Wash the green chilies thoroughly and dry them using a paper towel. You can choose to keep the chilies whole for a spicier kick, or you can slice them lengthwise and remove the seeds for a milder heat.

Sauté the Ingredients:
Heat the mustard oil in a pan over medium heat until it starts to smoke slightly. Add the minced garlic to the hot oil and sauté until it turns golden and aromatic. Add the chopped onions and sauté until they become translucent and lightly caramelized.

Cook the Green Chilies:
Add the green chilies to the pan and cook them until they start to blister and soften. You can adjust the cooking time based on how tender you want the chilies to be.

Mash and Season:
Using a mortar and pestle, a fork, or the back of a spoon, start mashing the cooked green chilies, onions, and garlic together. The goal is to create a coarse mash.

Adjust Seasoning:
Add salt to taste and continue mashing to mix the salt evenly throughout the mixture.

Add Lemon Juice:
Squeeze the juice from half a lemon into the chili mixture. The lemon juice adds a tangy flavor that complements the spiciness.

Final Mixing:
Mix all the ingredients together thoroughly, ensuring the flavors are well combined.

Serve Chilli Bhorta:
Chilli Bhorta is commonly served as a spicy condiment alongside rice and various curry dishes. It can also be served with bread, paratha, or other flatbreads to balance the heat.

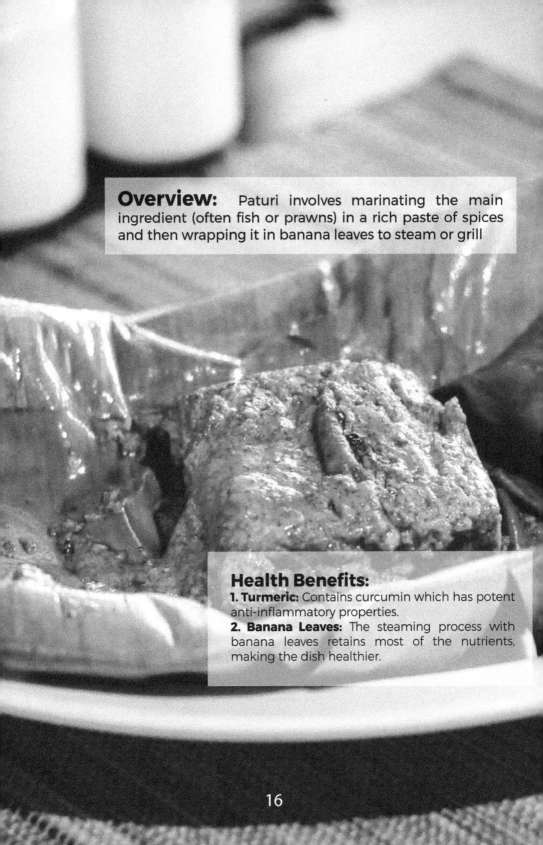

Overview: Paturi involves marinating the main ingredient (often fish or prawns) in a rich paste of spices and then wrapping it in banana leaves to steam or grill

Health Benefits:
1. Turmeric: Contains curcumin which has potent anti-inflammatory properties.
2. Banana Leaves: The steaming process with banana leaves retains most of the nutrients, making the dish healthier.

16

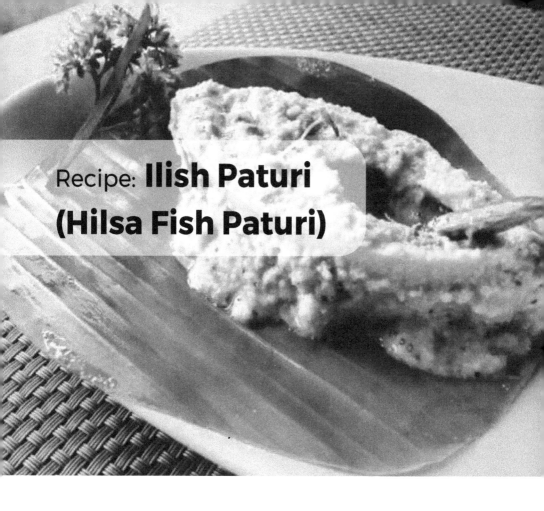

Recipe: **Ilish Paturi (Hilsa Fish Paturi)**

Ingredients:

pieces of Hilsa fish----------2
tbsp mustard paste----------2
tsp turmeric powder---------1
tsp red chilli powder---------1
Mustard oil
Salt to taste
Banana leaves for wrapping

Procedure:

1. Marinate the fish with mustard paste, turmeric, chilli powder, salt, and mustard oil.

2. Place each fish piece on a banana leaf, wrap, and secure with a string.

3. Steam or grill until cooked through.

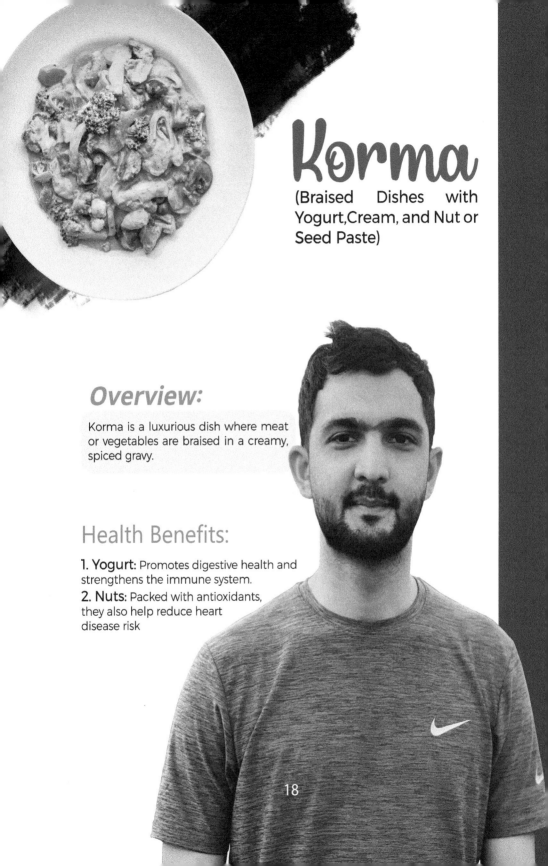

Korma

(Braised Dishes with Yogurt,Cream, and Nut or Seed Paste)

Overview:

Korma is a luxurious dish where meat or vegetables are braised in a creamy, spiced gravy.

Health Benefits:

1. Yogurt: Promotes digestive health and strengthens the immune system.

2. Nuts: Packed with antioxidants, they also help reduce heart disease risk

18

Chiken korma

Ingredients:

- 500g chicken pieces
- 1 cup yogurt
- 2 onions, finely sliced
- 2 tbsp cashew paste
- 1 tsp ginger-garlic paste
- 1 tsp turmeric, chilli, and cumin powder
- Salt to taste
- Ghee or oil for cooking

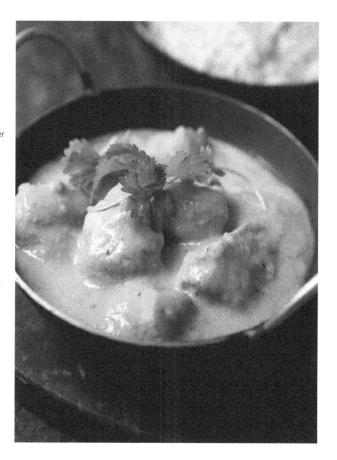

Procedure:

1. In a pan, fry the onions in ghee or oil until golden brown.

2. Add ginger-garlic paste, followed by the spice powders.

3. Add chicken pieces, yogurt, and cashew paste.

4. Cook until the chicken is tender and the gravy is rich and aromatic.

The magic of **Bangladeshi** cuisine lies in these traditional methods of harnessing the power of spices, not just for flavor, but for holistic well-being. Embracing these recipes means not only tantalizing the taste buds but also nourishing the body in a profound way.

Section 1.4: The Art of Roasting and Grinding Spices

Roasting and grinding spices at home is a tradition that is still upheld in many Bangladeshi hous holds. This process elevates the flavor of spices, and the freshly ground spice has a significantly superior flavor profile compared to store-bought versions.

In the heart of Bangladeshi cuisine lies its spices, freshly ground, roasted, and meticulously blended. This tradition of roasting and grinding spices at home, though it seems simple, plays a pivotal role in the complex and layered flavors synonymous with our dishes.

In conclusion, the spice trails of Bangladesh provide a deep and varied landscape that is integral to our cuisine. With an understanding of these spices, their origins, and uses, you'll be equipped to navigate this rich culinary tradition. In the next chapter, we will look at the essentials of Bangladeshi cuisine. Until then, let these spices stir your imagination and prepare you for the exciting journey ahead.

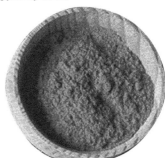

The Art *of* Roasting Spices

When spices are roasted, the heat draws out their essential oils, enriching their aroma and deepening their taste. This simple yet crucial step can transform an ordinary dish into an **extraordinary** one.

Health Benefits:

1. Activated Compounds: Roasting spices can activate certain beneficial compounds, increasing their potency.

2. Digestion Aid: Many roasted spices aid in digestion and have anti-inflammatory properties.

Recipe: **Homemade Garam Masala**

Ingredients:

 - 2 tbsp coriander seeds

 - 1 tbsp cumin seeds

 - 5-6 cloves

 - 1-inch cinnamon stick

 - 1 tsp fennel seeds

 - 5-6 green cardamom pods

 - 1 tsp black peppercorns

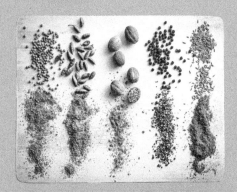

Procedure:

1. Dry roast each spice separately in a pan over low heat. Stir constantly until they release their aroma.
2. Let them cool down completely.
3. Grind them together in a mortar and pestle or a spice grinder until they form a fine powder.
4. Store in an airtight container.

The Importance of Freshly Ground Spices

The act of grinding spices right before their use ensures the retention of essential oils, which are often lost in pre-ground, store-bought versions. This not only provides a burst of flavor but also amplifies the health benefits associated with each spice.

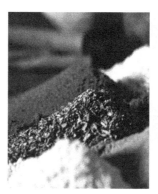

Health Benefits:

1. Essential Oils:
Freshly ground spices retain more essential oils, which are the heart of a spice's flavor and therapeutic properties.

2. No Additives:
Home-ground spices are free from additives and preservatives often found in commercial versions.

Recipe: Freshly Ground Turmeric Paste

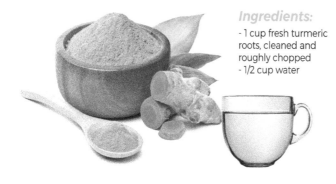

Ingredients:
- 1 cup fresh turmeric roots, cleaned and roughly chopped
- 1/2 cup water

Procedure:

1. Blend the turmeric roots with water until a smooth paste forms.

2. Store in a glass jar in the refrigerator. Use as required for curries, stews, or even in smoothies.

Concluding Thoughts

As we journey through Bangladeshi cuisine, the deep-rooted significance of spices becomes evident. It's not just about the taste; it's about the history, culture, and health interwoven with every grain of spice.With a solid grasp on these spices and their nuances, you're not only preparing to cook but to narrate stories of our rich heritage through your dishes.In the subsequent chapter, we will delve deeper into the cornerstones of Bangladeshi cuisine. But for now, let the enticing aromas of freshly roasted and ground spices guide your culinary explorations and whet your appetite for more.

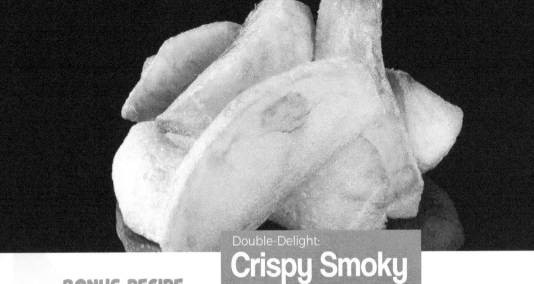

Double-Delight:
Crispy Smoky
Paprika Potatoes

Indulge in the crunch and flavor of our Crispy Smoky Paprika Potatoes! This dual-cooking method combines the best of baking and frying to deliver a spud sensation unlike any other. With the deep notes of smoked paprika and a hint of parsley freshness, these potatoes are set to be the star of any meal. Dive into our recipe below for a taste of crispy perfection!

Ingredients:

- Potatoes (preferably a starchy variety like Russet) - as many as you need
- Salt, to taste
- Smoked paprika, to taste
- Dried parsley, to taste
- Olive oil or your preferred cooking oil (for baking)
- Frying oil (like canola or vegetable oil)

Instructions:

1. Preparation:
- Wash the potatoes meticulously. For added texture and flavor, consider retaining the skins, but peeling is optional.
- Slice the potatoes uniformly to ensure even cooking.

2. Boil:
- Put the potatoes in a sizable pot, covering them with cold water and a dash of salt.
- Boil the water and allow the potatoes to cook just until they soften slightly. Depending on their size, this should take around 8-10 minutes.
- Drain and steam-dry the potatoes for a short while.

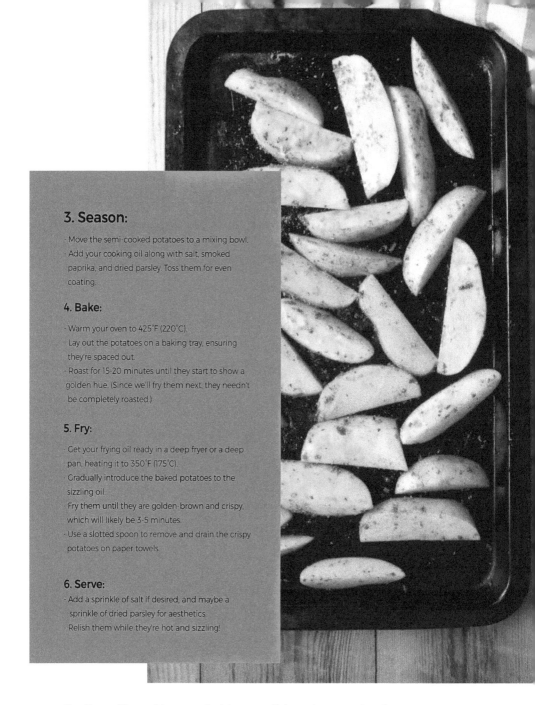

3. Season:

- Move the semi-cooked potatoes to a mixing bowl.
- Add your cooking oil along with salt, smoked
  paprika, and dried parsley. Toss them for even
  coating.

4. Bake:

- Warm your oven to 425°F (220°C).
- Lay out the potatoes on a baking tray, ensuring
  they're spaced out.
- Roast for 15-20 minutes until they start to show a
  golden hue. (Since we'll fry them next, they needn't
  be completely roasted.)

5. Fry:

- Get your frying oil ready in a deep fryer or a deep
  pan, heating it to 350°F (175°C).
- Gradually introduce the baked potatoes to the
  sizzling oil.
- Fry them until they are golden-brown and crispy,
  which will likely be 3-5 minutes.
- Use a slotted spoon to remove and drain the crispy
  potatoes on paper towels.

6. Serve:

- Add a sprinkle of salt if desired, and maybe a
  sprinkle of dried parsley for aesthetics.
- Relish them while they're hot and sizzling!

Bursting with smokiness and with a tantalizing crispy exterior, these potatoes are a treat for the senses. Perfect as a side dish or even a snack, their unique double-cooking method ensures a taste and texture that's hard to beat. Crispy on the outside, soft on the inside – dive in and *enjoy!*

A Crispy Delight with a Twist

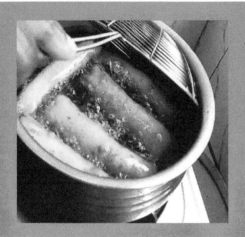

Journey along the riverside of flavor with **Arfatul's** signature tempura batter. Featuring the unique blend of pea flour, smoky paprika, and fragrant dried parsley, this recipe promises a crispy embrace to your favorite ingredients. Perfect for those serene evenings by the river or any festive gathering. Dive into the instructions below to create the perfect **tempura!**

Ingredients:

- 1 cup pea flour
- 1 1/4 cup ice-cold water (or soda water for extra crispiness)
- 1/2 teaspoon salt
- 1/2 teaspoon baking powder (optional, for - a lighter texture)
- 1 teaspoon smoked paprika
- 1 teaspoon dried parsley

Instructions:

- **Sifting:** Begin by sifting the pea flour, salt, baking powder (if you're incorporating it), smoked paprika, and dried parsley into a broad mixing vessel. This ensures you have a batter without clumps and spices that blend harmoniously.

- **Mixing:** Gradually introduce the ice-cold water (or soda water) to the sifted dry components, whisking as you go. Mix just until they blend; a few lumps are acceptable. Avoid overmixing, as it can result in a thick batter upon frying.

- **Chill:** Retain the batter's coldness for the best outcomes. Position the batter-filled bowl within a larger bowl filled with ice or use it straight after making.

- **Dipping & Frying:** Preheat your frying oil to about 350°F (175°C). Immerse your chosen items (like vegetables or seafood) into the batter, ensuring a consistent coat. Carefully set them into the boiling oil and fry till they're a golden hue.

- **Draining:** Once fried, extract the tempura pieces from the oil and place them on a cooling rack positioned over a baking sheet or on absorbent paper towels.

Tips:

- For the ultimate crispy outcome, always ensure your batter is cold and your oil is sufficiently hot.
- The incorporation of smoked paprika imparts a captivating reddish hue and a smoky undertone to the batter. In contrast, dried parsley introduces subtle green dots and a gentle herbaceous flavor.

Whether you're a seasoned chef or a **beginner**, this Riverside Tempura Embrace is sure to impress. Perfectly golden and crispy on the outside with a hint of smokiness and herbs, it's a treat not to be missed. **Happy frying!**

Mint Sauce

Dive into a burst of fresh flavors with our Mint and Coriander Sauce, enhanced with a sweet touch of Mango Chutney. This versatile dip combines the coolness of mint, the zing of coriander, and the creaminess of yogurt, perfect for grilled meats, snacks, or a tangy salad dressing. Follow our easy step-by-step recipe and elevate your meals to a gourmet experience!

Ingredients

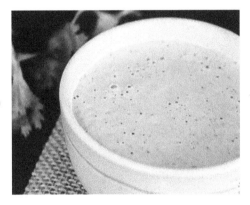

- 1 cup fresh mint leaves, packed
- 1 cup fresh coriander (cilantro) leaves, packed
- 1-2 green chilies (adjust to your heat preference)
- 2 tablespoons mango chutney
- 1/2 cup plain yogurt (Greek or regular, depending on your consistency preference)
- Salt, to taste
- 1 clove garlic

Instructions

Prepare Ingredients: Start by washing the mint and coriander leaves thoroughly. Remove any hard stems. Roughly chop the green chilies and garlic (you can remove the seeds from the chilies if you want it less spicy).

Blending: In a blender or food processor, combine the mint leaves, coriander leaves, green chilies, garlic, and mango chutney. Add a splash of water, if needed, and blend until you achieve a smooth paste.

Mix with Yogurt: Transfer the blended mixture to a bowl. Stir in the yogurt until you achieve a smooth consistency. If your sauce is too thick, you can add a little more yogurt or a splash of water to thin it out.

Flavoring: Taste the sauce and add salt according to your preference.

Serve: Transfer the sauce to a serving bowl. While it can be served immediately, letting it sit for a few hours (or overnight in the refrigerator) will allow the flavors to meld and enhance.

Storage: Store any leftovers in an airtight container in the refrigerator. Use within 3-4 days for the best taste and freshness.

Unleash the true potential of your meals with this tantalizing sauce. Perfect for **summer BBQs, cozy dinners**, or even as a spread for your sandwiches. *Enjoy!*

28

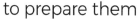

Bangladeshi cuisine, with its intricate layers of flavor, might seem complex to an outsider. However, at its heart, it is grounded on a few essential elements: **rice, fish, lentils, and vegetables.** In this chapter, we delve into the importance of these staples and the varied techniques used to prepare them

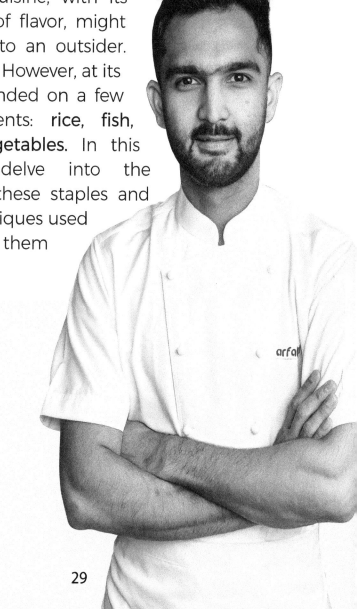

29

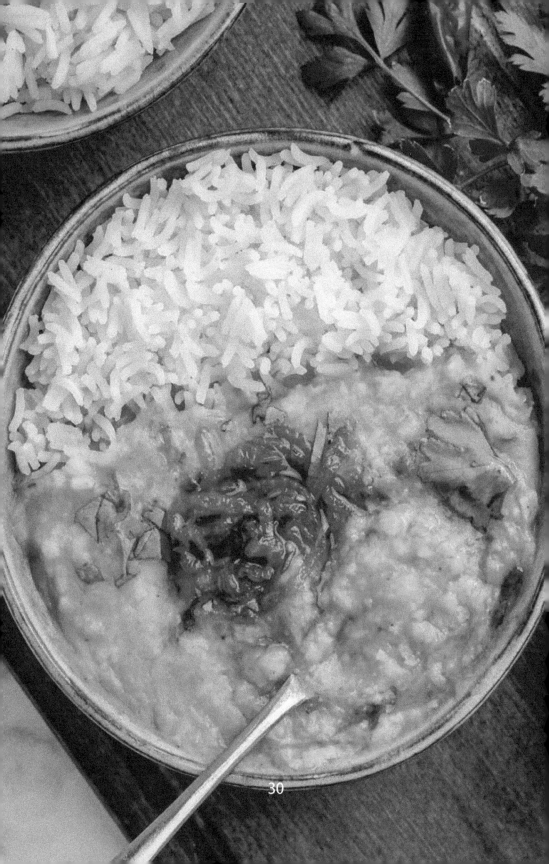

Rice-The Heart of the Meal

Rice, or 'Bhaat', is the cornerstone of Bangladeshi meals. Whether it's the everyday plain boiled rice, the fragrant 'polao', or the festive biryanis, rice dishes are diverse and versatile. *The most commonly* used rice variety is parboiled rice, known for its unique texture and nutty flavor. Other varieties such as 'Kalijira', 'Chinigura', and 'Kataribhog' are used for special dishes due to their unique aroma and flavors. *The methods of cooking* rice range from boiling to steaming, and each method has its distinct effect on the texture and taste of the rice.

Plain Boiled Rice
(Bhaat)

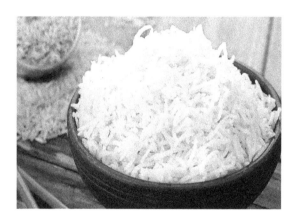

Ingredients:

- 1-------- cup parboiled rice
- 2 ---------------- cups water
- 1 ---------------------tsp salt

Instructions:

1. Rinse the rice under cold water until the water runs clear.

2. Add the rice, water, and salt to a pot.

3. Bring to a boil over medum-high heat.

4. Once boiling, reduce the heat to low, cover the pot, and let it simmer for 15-20 minutes until all the water is absorbed and the rice is tender.

5. Fluff with a fork before serving.

Section 2.2:
Fish – The Soul of the Cuisine

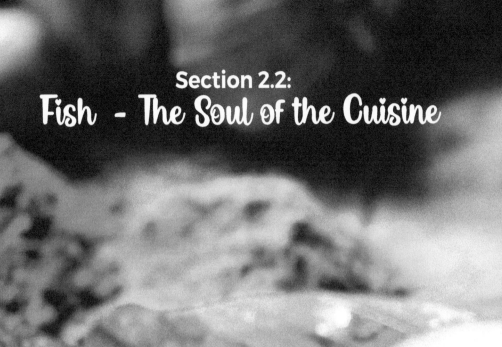

Bangladesh, the land of rivers, has an abundance of freshwater fish. Therefore, it's not surprising that fish, or 'Maach', is an integral part of Bangladeshi cuisine. From 'Hilsa' (Ilish), the national fish, to **'Rui' (Rohu), 'Katla', and 'Pabda'**, the varieties are endless.

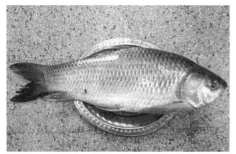

Fish is prepared in numerous ways - fried, grilled, or used in curries. One of the most popular methods is cooking fish in mustard sauce, known as 'Shorshe Maach'.

(SHORSHE MAACH)

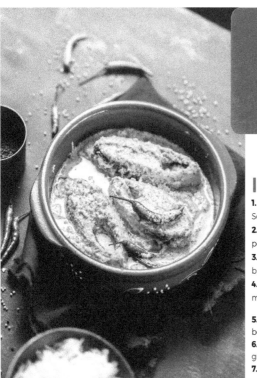

Ingredients:

- **500g**	Rohu fish, cut into pieces
- **2**	tbsp mustard seeds
- **1**	tsp turmeric powder
- **2**	green chillies
	Salt to taste
- **3**	tbsp mustard oil

Instructions:

1. Marinate the fish with salt and 1/2 tsp turmeric powder. Set aside for 15 minutes.

2. Make a paste with the mustard seeds, 1/2 tsp turmeric powder, 1 green chilli, and a little water.

3. Heat mustard oil in a pan. Fry the fish until golden brown and set aside.

4. In the same oil, add the mustard paste. Cook for a few minutes.

5. Add water as required, followed by salt. Bring it to a boil.

6. Add the fried fish and cook until done. Garnish with slit green chillies.

7. Serve hot with rice.

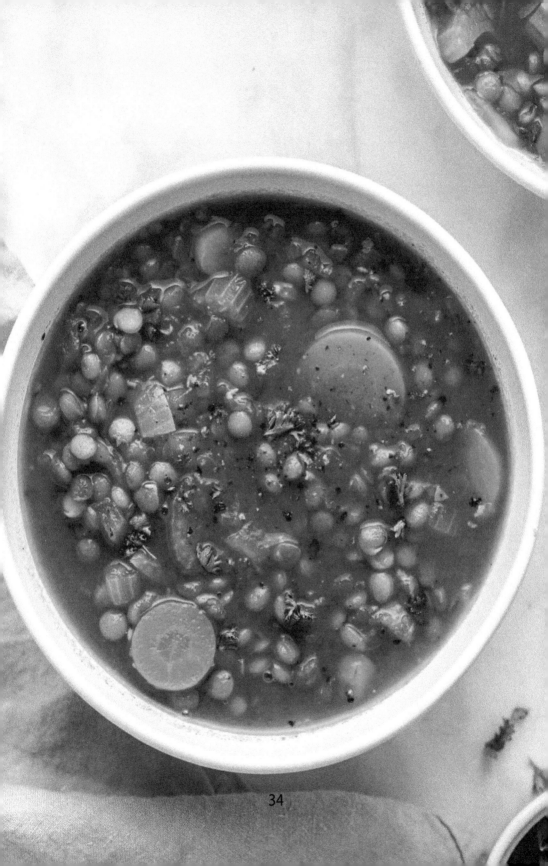

Section 2.3:

Lentils - A Bowl of Comfort

Lentils, or 'Dal', is the comfort food of Bangladesh. The most common lentil dish is 'Moshur Dal', made from red lentils. **The process is simple yet yields a flavorful result:** lentils are boiled with turmeric and salt, and then tempered with fried onions, garlic, and sometimes, additional spices. Lentils are served as a side dish and provide a balance to the spicy main dishes.

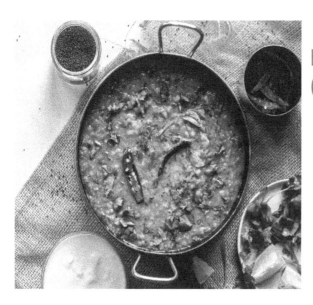

Red Lentil Dal (Moshur Dal)

Ingredients:
- 1 ....cup red lentils
- 1 ....tsp turmeric powder
- ....Salt to taste
- 2 ....tbsp oil
- 1 .... onion, finely chopped
- 2 ....cloves garlic, minced

Instructions:

1. Rinse the lentils under cold water until the water runs clear.
2. In a pot, add lentils, turmeric, salt, and 3 cups of water. Bring it to a boil.

3. Reduce the heat to low, cover the pot, and let it simmer until the lentils are soft.
4. In a separate pan, heat the oil and fry the onions until golden brown.

5. Add the minced garlic and cook for another minute.
6. Pour this tempering over the cooked lentils and mix well.
7. Serve hot with rice.

Vegetables -The Colorful Side

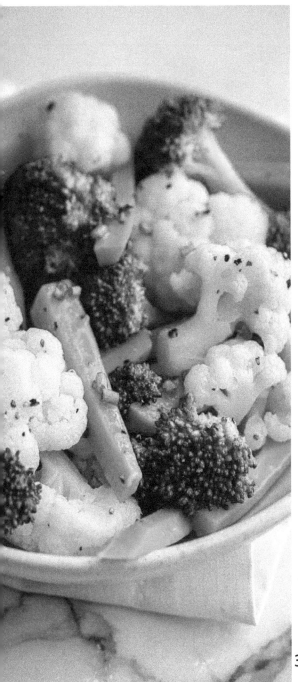

Bangladeshi cuisine boasts a wide array of vegetable dishes, known as 'Torkari'. From leafy greens to root vegetables and gourds, the variety is astounding.

Vegetables can be prepared in many ways: stir-fried, cooked into curries, or mashed into 'Bhorta'. One common feature is the use of 'Panch Phoron', a five-spice blend, to temper the dishes and add a unique flavor profile.

Bangladeshi cuisine is rooted in these essential ingredients, and each lends a different character to the dish. By understanding these staples, we can better appreciate the breadth and depth of the recipes that follow.As we delve into the recipes in subsequent chapters,we will further explore how these elements come

together to form delicious, hearty meals that are the hallmark of Bangladeshi cuisine.

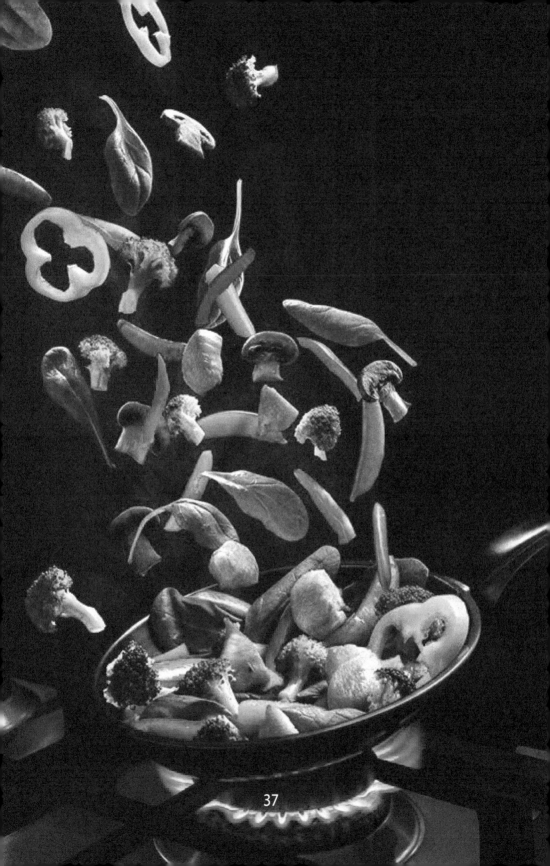

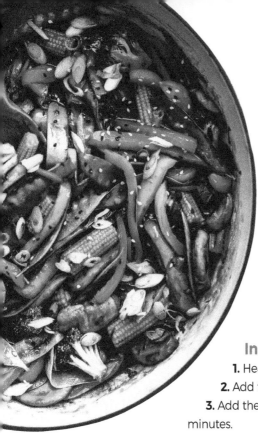

Stir-Fried Vegetables (Torkari)

Ingredients:
- 1 cup mixed vegetables (like carrot, beans, bell peppers)
- 1 tsp Panch Phoron (equal parts of fenugreek seed, nigella seed, cumin seed, black mustard seed, and fennel seed)
- 2 tbsp oil
- Salt to taste

Instructions:
1. Heat oil in a pan.
2. Add the Panch Phoron and let it crackle.
3. Add the mixed vegetables and stir fry for a few minutes.
4. Add salt, cover the pan, and cook on low heat until the vegetables are tender.
5. Serve hot with rice and dal.

Enjoy cooking these quintessential Bangladeshi dishes!

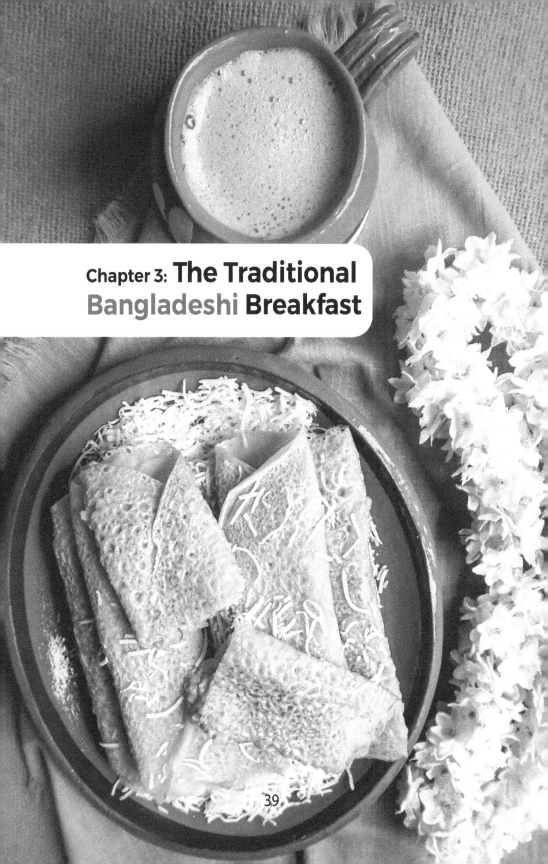

Chapter 3: **The Traditional Bangladeshi Breakfast**

Breakfast is an important meal in **Bangladeshi cuisine**, one that is steeped in tradition and culture. It is hearty and varied, designed to fuel you for the day ahead. In this chapter, we explore the delights of a traditional Bangladeshi breakfast.

Section 3.1:
Pitha - The Versatile Breakfast Snack

Pitha is a broad category of rice-based snacks or desserts that are popular for breakfast. These come in a wide variety, such as 'Bhapa Pitha' (steamed rice cakes), 'Chitoi Pitha' (rice pancakes), and 'Puli Pitha' (sweet dumplings), each having a unique taste and texture.

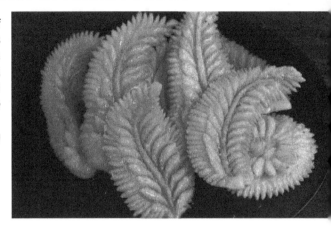

Bhapa Pitha (Steamed Rice Cake)

Ingredients:
- **1** ----------------------cup rice flour
- **1/2**------------cup coconut, grated
- **1/2**----------------------cup jaggery

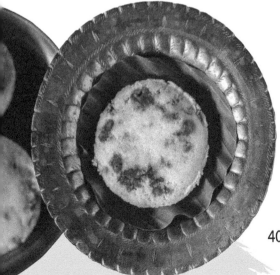

Instructions:
1. Make a dough by gradually adding warm water to the rice flour. The dough should be firm but pliable.
2. Make a filling by mixing the grated coconut and jaggery.
3. Form the dough into a small bowl, fill it with the coconut-jaggery mix, and seal it.
4. Place each pitha in a steamer and steam for **10-15** minutes.
5. Serve warm.

Paratha and Bhaji

A common and filling breakfast option is 'Paratha' (flaky, pan-fried bread) served with 'Bhaji' (a spicy stirfried vegetable or meat dish). The paratha can also be served with dal or eggs, making it a versatile dish that can be varied according to preference.

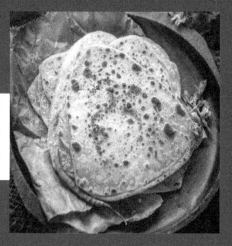

Paratha and Cabbage-Potato Bhaji

Paratha Ingredients:

- 2   cups wheat flour
-                      Water
-                       Salt
-       Ghee (clarified butter)

Cabbage-Potato Bhaji Ingredients:

2 potatoes, diced
Half a head of cabbage, finely shredded
1 onion, chopped
2 green chilies, chopped
1 tsp turmeric powder
Salt
Oil
1 tsp cumin seeds (optional for added flavor)
1/2 tsp red chili powder (optional for added spice)

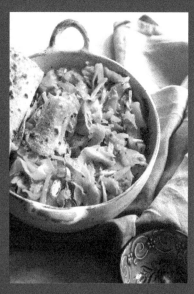

Instructions:

For Paratha:

a. Make a firm dough with the wheat flour, water, salt, and a touch of ghee.
b. Divide the dough into balls and roll each into a flat round shape.
c. Cook each paratha on a hot griddle, applying ghee on both sides until golden brown.

For Cabbage-Potato Bhaji:

a. Heat oil in a pan. If using cumin seeds, add them first and let them sizzle for a few seconds.
b. Add the chopped onions and green chilies. Sauté until the onions become translucent.
c. Add the diced potatoes and cook for a few minutes until they start to brown slightly.
d. Add the shredded cabbage, turmeric powder, salt, and red chili powder (if using). Mix well.
e. Cover the pan and let the vegetables cook on a low flame, stirring occasionally. The moisture from the cabbage should help cook the potatoes. If needed, sprinkle a little water to prevent sticking.
f. Continue to cook until the potatoes are soft and the cabbage is well-cooked.

Serve the parathas hot with the cabbage-potato bhaji on the side.

Section 3.3: Halwa-Puri

For those with a sweet tooth, 'Halwa-Puri' is a delightful choice. 'Puri' is a type of deep-fried bread, often served with 'Halwa', a sweet dish made from semolina or carrots.

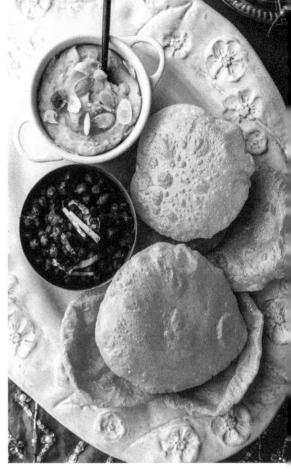

Halwa-Puri

Puri Ingredients:
- 1   cup wheat flour
- Water
- Salt
- Oil for frying

Halwa Ingredients:
- 1 cup semolina
- 1 cup sugar
- 4 cups water
- 4 tbsp ghee
- 1/2 cup mixed dry fruits

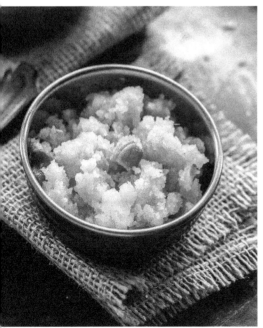

Instructions:
1. Make a firm dough with the wheat flour, water, and salt.
2. Roll the dough into small, flat rounds and deep fry in hot oil until puffed and golden.
3. For the halwa, heat ghee in a pan. Add the semolina and roast until golden.
4. Boil the water and sugar in a separate pot. Gradually add this to the roasted semolina, stirring
constantly to avoid lumps.
5. Add the dry fruits and cook until the halwa leaves the sides of the pan.
6. Serve the puris with the hot halwa.

Section 3.4: **Kichuri**

'Kichuri', a hearty dish made from rice and lentils, is often eaten for breakfast, especially during the rainy season. It is usually served with fried Hilsa fish or a variety of pickles.

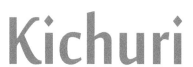

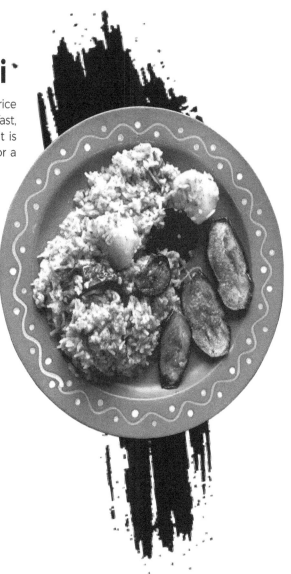

Ingredients:

cup rice --- 1
cup red lentils --------------------------- 1/2
onion, chopped ---------------------------- 1
green chilies ------------------------------ 2
tsp turmeric powder --------------------- 1
Salt
tbsp oil ------------------------------------- 2

Instructions:

1. Wash the rice and lentils together and set aside.
2. Heat oil in a pot. Add the onions and green chilies. Saute until the onions are golden.
3. Add the rice and lentils, turmeric, and salt. Stir well.
4. Add water and bring it to a boil.
5. Reduce the heat, cover the pot, and let it simmer until both the rice and lentils are cooked.
6. Serve hot with pickle or fried fish.

Section 3.5:
TEA - THE PERFECT COMPANION

No breakfast is complete without a steaming cup of tea, or 'cha'. Tea in Bangladesh is usually black, strongly brewed, and served with milk and sugar. It's the perfect companion to any breakfast dish and a great way to start the day.

Tea (Cha)

These are just a few examples of the diverse breakfast options in Bangladeshi cuisine. Each dish offers a unique combination of flavors and ingredients, ensuring that every morning can be a new culinary adventure. In the following chapters, we will explore the wide variety of dishes that make up lunch and dinner in Bangladeshi cuisine. Until then, happy breakfasting!

The Health
Essence of Cha

Tea, especially when consumed without an excess of sugar, has several health benefits:

1. Antioxidants: Tea is rich in catechins, which are natural antioxidants that help in preventing cell damage and reducing inflammation.

2. Heart Health: Regular consumption of tea can be linked to a reduced risk of heart diseases. It can help in regulating cholesterol levels and improving blood pressure.

3. Mental Alertness: The caffeine content, though less than in coffee, is sufficient to promote alertness. Additionally, it contains an amino acid called L-theanine, which has a calming effect and, when combined with caffeine, can help improve brain function.

5. Oral Health: The tannins present in tea can suppress the growth of bacteria in the mouth, potentially reducing the risk of cavities.

4. Metabolism and Fat Burn: Tea can help in boosting metabolic rates, which may promote fat burning in the short term.

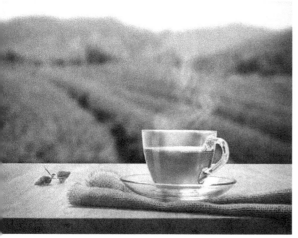

Ingredients:

- 1 ---------------------------------cup water
- 1 ------------------------------tsp tea leaves
- ------------------------------Sugar to taste
- 1/2 --------------------------------cup milk

Instructions:

1. Boil water in a pot.
2. Add the tea leaves and let it boil for a minute.
3. Add the sugar and milk. Bring it to a boil.
4. Strain the tea into a cup and serve hot.

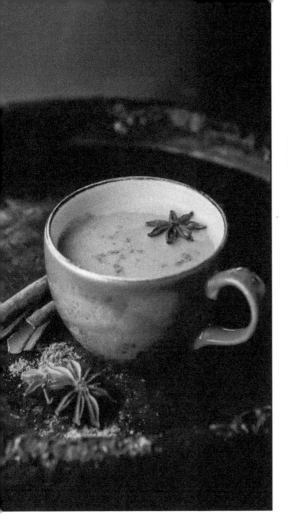

Masala Cha (Spiced Tea)

Give your regular tea a twist with a sprinkle of spices, not just for flavor but also for added health benefits.

Ingredients:

- 1 cup water
- 1 tsp tea leaves
- Sugar to taste
- 1/2 cup milk
- 1 cardamom pod, crushed
- 1 small cinnamon stick
- 1 clove
- A pinch of ground ginger

Instructions:

1. Boil water in a pot with the cardamom, cinnamon, clove, and ginger.

2. Once the water takes on a slight color from the spices, add the tea leaves and let it boil for a minute.

3. Add sugar according to preference.
4. Pour in the milk and bring the tea to a boil again.
5. Strain the masala cha into a cup, leaving behind the spices, and serve hot.

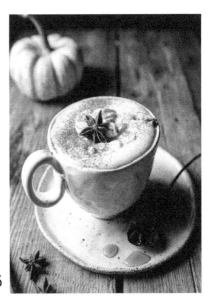

Lemon Ginger Cha

An uplifting version of the traditional tea, this recipe is perfect for those under the weather or just looking for a refreshing twist

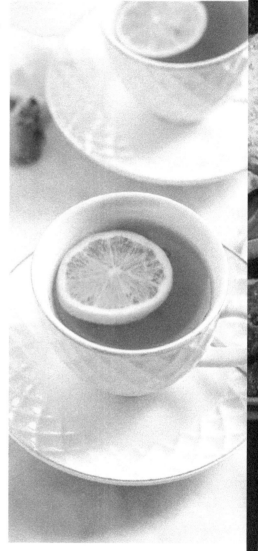

Ingredients:

- **1** ....cup water
- **1** ....tsp tea leaves
- - ....Honey or sugar to taste
- - ....Juice of half a lemon
- **1** ....-inch ginger, crushed

Instructions:

1. Boil water in a pot with the crushed ginger.

2. Add the tea leaves and allow it to simmer for a minute.

3. Add honey or sugar according to your taste.

4. Strain the tea into a cup, add the freshly squeezed lemon juice, stir, and serve hot.

Concluding Note

The world of Bangladeshi tea is as vast as its lush tea gardens. While the standard milk tea holds its own special place, there are countless variations to explore. As you sip on your Cha, remember that you're not just consuming a beverage, but partaking in a ritual that holds within its depths centuries of tradition, health benefits, and stories untold.

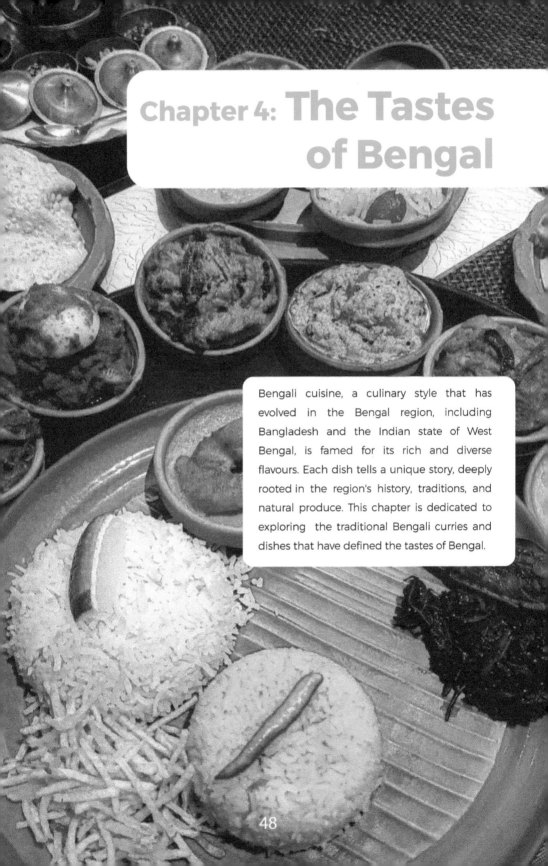

Chapter 4: The Tastes of Bengal

Bengali cuisine, a culinary style that has evolved in the Bengal region, including Bangladesh and the Indian state of West Bengal, is famed for its rich and diverse flavours. Each dish tells a unique story, deeply rooted in the region's history, traditions, and natural produce. This chapter is dedicated to exploring the traditional Bengali curries and dishes that have defined the tastes of Bengal.

Section 4.1: **Hilsa Delights**

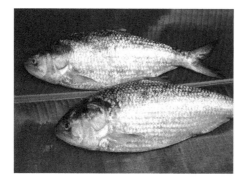

'Hilsa', or 'Ilish', the national fish of Bangladesh, is celebrated in numerous dishes that capture the essence of Bengal. The most beloved among these is 'Ilish Bhapa', or steamed hilsa, where the fish is marinated in a paste of mustard and green chillies, wrapped in banana leaves, and then steamed to perfection.

Ilish Bhapa (Steamed Hilsa)

Ingredients:

- **500g** Hilsa fish
- **2** tbsp mustard seeds
- **4-5** green chilies
- **1/2** tsp turmeric powder
- Salt to taste
- **4** tbsp mustard oil
- Banana leaves for wrapping

Instructions:

1. Clean and wash the Hilsa fish. Set it aside.
2. Make a paste of mustard seeds, green chilies, turmeric, and salt in a grinder.
3. Coat the fish pieces with the mustard paste.
4. Drizzle mustard oil over the fish.
5. Wrap each piece of fish in banana leaves and steam for about 15-20 minutes.
6. Serve hot with steamed rice.

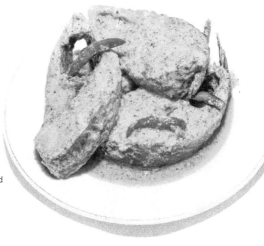

Section 4.2: Traditional Curries

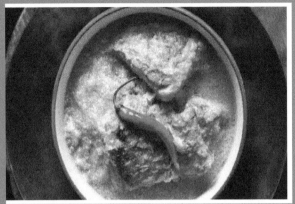

Bengal boasts an array of curries, each with its unique blend of spices. 'Doi Maach' is a classic fish curry with a yogurt-based gravy, offering a delightful tanginess. 'Murgir Jhol', a chicken curry, and 'Kosha Mangsho', a rich mutton curry, are meat-based favourites with deeply flavourful gravies.

Doi Maach
(Fish Curry in Yogurt Sauce)

Ingredients:

- 500g Rohu fish
- 2 onions, finely chopped
- 1 cup yogurt
- 1 tsp turmeric powder
- 1 tsp red chili powder
- Salt to taste
- 4 tbsp mustard oil

Instructions:

1. Marinate the fish with turmeric and salt.
2. Heat oil in a pan and fry the fish until golden. Set aside.
3. In the same pan, fry the onions until golden.
4. Add the yogurt, turmeric, chili powder, and salt. Cook until the oil separates.
5. Add the fried fish and some water. Simmer for 10-15 minutes.
6. Serve hot with rice.

50

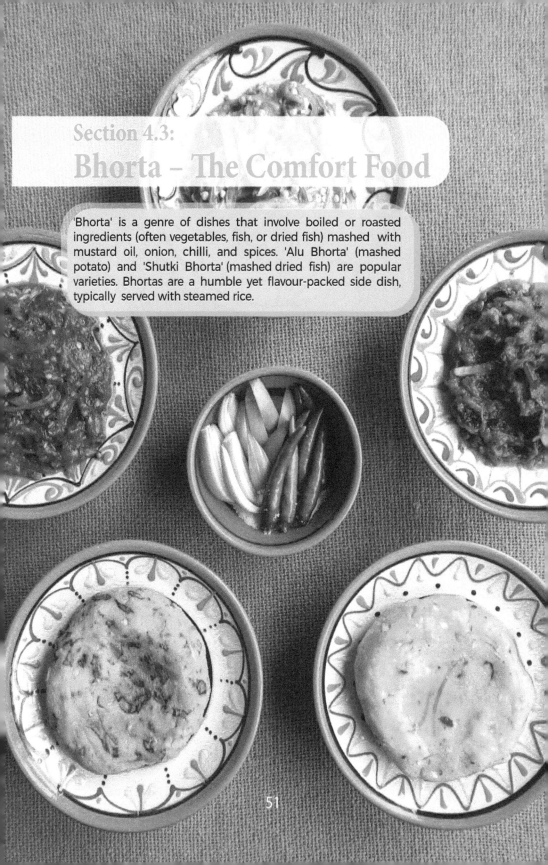

Bhorta – The Comfort Food

'Bhorta' is a genre of dishes that involve boiled or roasted ingredients (often vegetables, fish, or dried fish) mashed with mustard oil, onion, chilli, and spices. 'Alu Bhorta' (mashed potato) and 'Shutki Bhorta' (mashed dried fish) are popular varieties. Bhortas are a humble yet flavour-packed side dish, typically served with steamed rice.

Shutki Bhorta

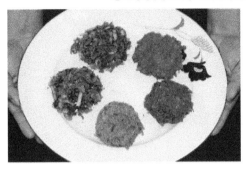

also known as "Dried Fish Mash," is a popular Bangladeshi dish that is full of bold flavors. It's made from dried fish, often referred to as "shutki" in Bengali, which is mashed and combined with various spices and ingredients. Here's a basic recipe for making Shutki Bhorta:

Ingredients:

- Dried fish (shutki): 200 grams
- Onion: 1 medium, finely chopped
- Green chilies: 2-3 (adjust according to your spice preference), finely chopped
- Garlic: 3-4 cloves, minced
- Mustard oil: 2-3 tablespoons
- Salt: to taste
- Red chili powder: 1/2 teaspoon (adjust according to your spice preference)
- Coriander leaves: A handful, chopped (optional)
- Lemon juice: From half a lemon

Instructions:

1. Prepare the Dried Fish:
- Begin by soaking the dried fish in warm water for about 15-20 minutes. This helps soften the fish and removes excess salt.
- After soaking, rinse the fish thoroughly under running water to remove any remaining salt and debris.

2. Cook the Dried Fish:
- In a pot, add the soaked and rinsed dried fish and enough water to cover it.
- Bring the water to a boil and let the fish cook for about 15-20 minutes, or until it becomes soft and easily flakes apart.
- Once cooked, drain the water and let the fish cool down.

3. Mash the Dried Fish:
- Once the fish is cool enough to handle, use your hands to remove the bones and separate the flesh from the skin.
- Mash the fish using your fingers or a fork until it reaches a shredded consistency.

4. Prepare the Bhorta:
- Heat mustard oil in a pan over medium heat until it starts to smoke a little. This helps remove the pungent taste of raw mustard oil.
- Add the minced garlic and chopped green chilies to the hot oil. Sauté them until the garlic turns golden and fragrant.

5. Add the Ingredients:
- Add the chopped onions to the pan and sauté until they become translucent and slightly caramelized.

6. Add the Dried Fish:
- Add the mashed dried fish to the pan and mix it well with the sautéed onions, garlic, and chilies.

7. Seasoning:
- Sprinkle red chili powder and salt over the mixture. Adjust the amount of chili powder according to your taste preference.

8. Mash and Cook:
- Use a spatula or the back of a spoon to mash and mix the ingredients together. Keep mashing and mixing until everything is well combined and the flavors meld together.

9. Finish and Serve:
- Add a squeeze of lemon juice and chopped coriander leaves to the mixture. Mix well.
- Taste and adjust the seasoning if needed.

10. Serve Shutki Bhorta:
- Shutki Bhorta is traditionally served with steamed rice as a flavorful side dish. You can also enjoy it with flatbreads.

Section 4.4:

Dhaka's Bakarkhani

'Bakarkhani' is a thick, spiced flat -bread, originating from the old Dhaka region. Sweet and savoury at the same time, it is traditionally served with tea, and has a unique texture that sets it apart from other breads.

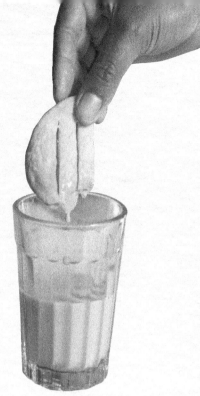

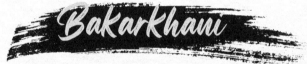

Ingredients:
- 2   cups all-purpose flour
- 1/2   cup ghee (clarified butter)
- 1/2   cup sugar
- 1/2   cup milk
- 1/4   tsp salt

Instructions:
1. In a large bowl, mix the flour, ghee, sugar, and salt.
2. Gradually add the milk and knead to make a dough.
3. Roll out the dough and fold it multiple times to create layers.

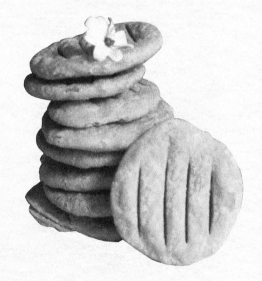

4. Roll out again into a thick flatbread.
5. Cook on a hot griddle until golden on both sides.
6. Serve hot with tea

Section 4.5:
Chotpoti, Fuchka and Bhel Puri – The Street Food Favourites

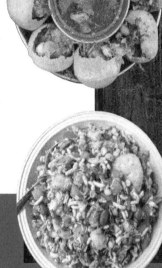

'Chotpoti' and 'Fuchka' are two beloved street foods in Bengal. 'Chotpoti' is a spicy and tangy chickpea curry, served with boiled eggs and a variety of chutneys. 'Fuchka', known as 'Pani Puri' in other parts of South Asia, is a hollow crispy ball filled with tamarind water, chickpeas, and spices.

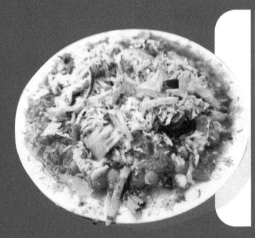

Each dish in the Bengali culinary repertoire provides a unique window into the region's rich cultural and culinary heritage. Through these traditional dishes, one can savour the tastes of Bengal and appreciate the complex layers of flavours that define this cuisine. As we progress through the book, we will delve deeper into specific types of dishes, revealing more culinary treasures of Bangladeshi cuisine.

Chotpoti

Ingredients:

- -cup dried peas — 1
- -boiled eggs — 2
- -onion, finely chopped — 1
- -green chilies, finely chopped — 2
- Tamarind chutney
- -Green chutney
- -Chaat masala
- -Salt to taste

Instructions:

1. Soak the peas overnight. Boil until soft.
2. Mix the boiled peas with onions, chilies, tamarind chutney, green chutney, chaat masala, and salt.
3. Garnish with boiled eggs and serve.

Fuchka

Fuchka, also known as Phuchka or Puchka in some regions of India, is a popular street food snack in Bangladesh and India. It's a hollow, crispy puri filled with a spicy mixture of tamarind water, chickpeas, and potatoes. Here's a basic recipe for making Bangladeshi Fuchka:

Ingredients:

For the Fuchka shells (puri):

1. 1 cup semolina (sooji)
2. A pinch of baking soda
3. Water (as needed)
4. Salt (a pinch)
5. Oil (for frying)

For the filling:

1. 2 large potatoes, boiled and mashed

2. 1/2 cup cooked white peas or chickpeas

3. 1-2 green chilies, finely chopped (adjust according to your spice tolerance)

4. A handful of chopped coriander leaves

5. 1/2 tsp roasted cumin powder

6. 1/2 tsp red chili powder

7. 1/2 tsp black salt

8. Salt to taste

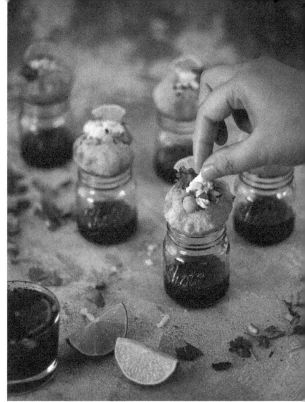

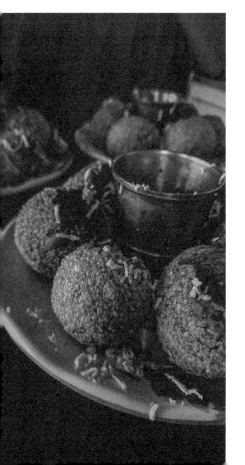

For the Tamarind water
(*optional but recommended*):

1. A ball of tamarind (lime-sized)

2. 2 cups of water

3. Black salt to taste

4. Roasted cumin powder

5. Green chili paste or red chili powder to taste

57

Instructions:

For the Fuchka shells (puri)

1. In a bowl, combine semolina, salt, and baking soda. Slowly add water, kneading as you go, to make a stiff dough. The consistency is vital; it should not be too soft.

2. Cover the dough with a damp cloth and let it rest for 15-20 minutes.

3. Make small marble-sized balls from the dough.

4. On a lightly oiled surface, roll each ball into a thin disc. Try to roll it as thin as possible without tearing.

5. Heat oil in a deep frying pan. Once it's hot, fry each disc until they puff up and turn golden brown. Remove and place on paper towels to remove excess oil.

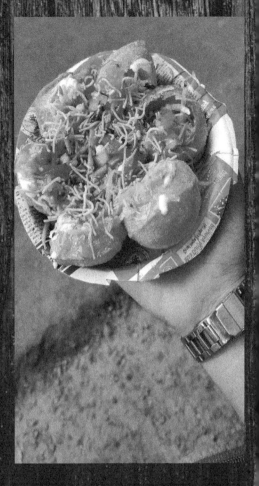

For the filling:

1. Mix mashed potatoes, chickpeas, green chilies, coriander leaves, cumin powder, red chili powder, black salt, and regular salt. Mix well and adjust the seasonings according to your preference.

1. Soak the tamarind ball in water for about an hour. Then, squeeze out the pulp, and strain it to get a watery consistency.

2. Add black salt, roasted cumin powder, and chili to taste. Mix well.

To serve:

1. Make a hole in the center of each Fuchka shell.

2. Fill it with the spicy potato filling.

3. Dip or pour some tamarind water into the filled Fuchka and enjoy immediately.

Remember, Fuchka is best enjoyed freshly made and consumed immediately to maintain its crispy texture. Adjust the spiciness and tanginess according to your preference. Enjoy your homemade Bangladeshi Fuchka!

Bhel Puri

Bhel Puri is a popular Indian street food, often associated with Mumbai, but it has many variations across different regions, including Bangladesh. The Bangladeshi variation might have some regional touches, but the essence is similar.

Here's a basic Bhel Puri recipe with a general South Asian touch:

Ingredients:

1. Puffed rice - **2** cups
2. Thin sev (crispy chickpea flour noodles) - **½** cup
3. Papdi (crispy flat puris) - **8-10,** crushed
4. Boiled potatoes - **1,** diced
5. Tomatoes - **1**, finely chopped 6. Onions - **1**, finely chopped
7. Cucumber - **½**, finely chopped (optional)

8. Green chilies - **1-2,** finely chopped (adjust according to heat preference)
9. Tamarind pulp - **3** tablespoons
10. Green chutney (mint and coriander) - **2** tablespoons
11. Red chili powder - **½** teaspoon
12. Roasted cumin powder - **½** teaspoon
13. Chaat masala - **1** teaspoon

14. Lemon juice - **1** tablespoon
15. Fresh coriander leaves - a handful, chopped
16. Raw mango - a few pieces, finely chopped (optional, if in season)
17. Peanuts - a handful, roasted
18. Salt - to taste

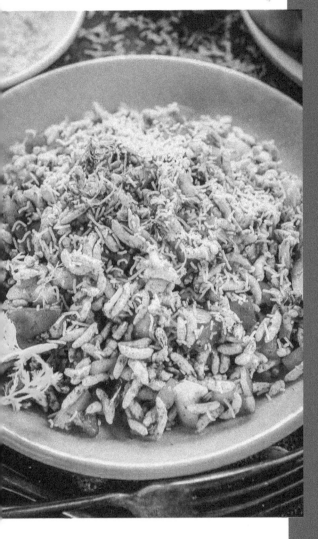

Instructions:

1. Tamarind Chutney: Mix the tamarind pulp with some water, sugar, and a pinch of salt. Boil it until you get a sauce-like consistency. Adjust the sweetness and tanginess according to your preference. Let it cool.

2. In a large mixing bowl, add the puffed rice, sev, and crushed papdi.
3. Add the chopped boiled potatoes, onions, tomatoes, cucumber, green chilies, and raw mango (if using).

4. Add the green chutney and tamarind chutney to the mixture. Mix well.

5. Sprinkle red chili powder, roasted cumin powder, chaat masala, and salt. Mix again.

6. Squeeze the lemon juice over the mixture and give it a final mix.

7. Top the Bhel Puri with some more sev, roasted peanuts, and chopped coriander leaves.

8. Serve immediately to retain the crunchiness.

Note: Adjust the spice levels according to your preference. Also, you can include or omit ingredients based on what's available or your personal liking. The key is the balance of flavors and textures, with the mixture of crunchy, soft, spicy, tangy, and sweet components.

Chapter 5:

The Feast of Biryani

Biryani, a one-pot dish of aromatic rice, tender meat, and fragrant spices, is considered a symbol of celebration in Bangladeshi cuisine. Though its origins are traced back to the Mughal Empire, it has been embraced and adapted by Bangladesh, leading to a variety of regional versions. In this chapter, we delve into the intricate world of biryani, from traditional classics to innovative variations.

Section 5.1: The Classic: Kacchi Biryani

Kacchi Biryani is considered the crown jewel of Bangladeshi cuisine. It's a layered dish made with partially cooked meat and partially cooked rice, which are then cooked together. The meat, usually mutton or chicken, is marinated overnight in a mix of yogurt, ginger, garlic, and special biryani spices before being layered with rice in a handi (heavy-bottomed pot), and then slow-cooked until done..

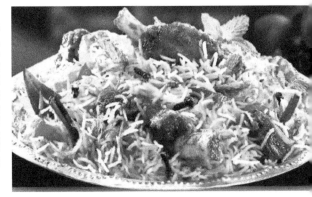

Kacchi Biryani Recipe

Ingredients:

- **1 kg** mutton (cut into pieces)
- **2 cups** basmati rice
- **1 cup** plain yogurt
- 2 tablespoons ginger paste
- 2 tablespoons garlic paste
- 2 tablespoons Biryani masala
- 1 large onion (finely sliced)
- 4 green chillies
- 1/2 cup ghee (clarified butter)
- Salt to taste
- A handful of fresh mint and coriander leaves
- 1 teaspoon saffron strands
  (soaked in 2 tablespoons warm milk)

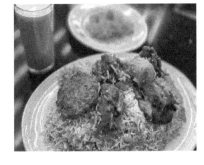
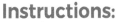
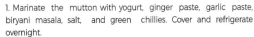

Instructions:

1. Marinate the mutton with yogurt, ginger paste, garlic paste, biryani masala, salt, and green chillies. Cover and refrigerate overnight.
2. Rinse the basmati rice under cold water until the water runs clear. Soak the rice in water for 30 minutes, then drain.
3. In a heavy-bottomed pot, heat the ghee over medium heat. Add the sliced onion and fry until they are golden brown.
4. Layer the marinated mutton over the onions, then layer the soaked and drained rice on top of the mutton.
5. Sprinkle the top with mint, coriander leaves, and saffron milk.
6. Cover the pot with a tight-fitting lid and cook on a low flame for about 2-3 hours, until the mutton is tender and the flavors have melded together.
7. Fluff the rice gently with a fork before serving.

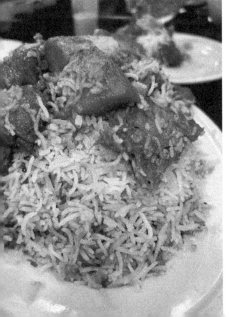

Section 5.2: The Everyday: Tehari

Tehari is a variant of biryani that is often cooked at home. It is less rich than the traditional biryani and usually made with beef. The process involves cooking the meat and rice together with the spices, making it a simpler and quicker version to prepare.

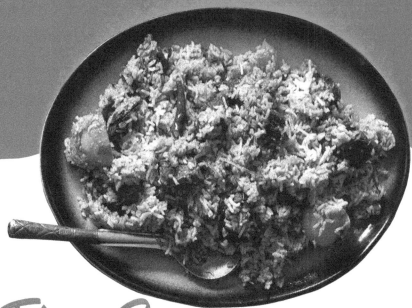

Tehari Recipe

Ingredients:

- 500g beef (cut into pieces)
- 2 cups basmati rice
- 1 large onion (finely sliced)
- 2 tablespoons ginger-garlic paste
- 2 tablespoons Tehari masala
- 1/2 cup vegetable oil
- Salt to taste
- 4 green chillies
- A handful of fresh coriander leaves

Instructions:

1. Rinse the basmati rice under cold water until the water runs clear. Soak the rice in water for 30 minutes,
then drain.
2. Heat the oil in a large pot over medium heat. Add the onion and fry until golden brown.
3. Add the beef, ginger-garlic paste, Tehari masala, salt, and green chillies to the pot. Stir well to coat the beef with the spices.
4. Add the drained rice to the pot and mix well.
5. Add enough water to cover the rice and beef, bring to a boil.
6. Once boiling, reduce the heat to low, cover the pot, and let it simmer for about 30-40 minutes, or until
the rice is cooked and the beef is tender.
7. Garnish with fresh coriander leaves before serving.

MOROG POLAO (CHICKEN PILAF)

Morog Polao is a treasured dish from Dhaka, the capital city of Bangladesh. It is often made during special occasions and festivities. This dish is a beautiful medley of succulent chicken pieces with aromatic rice. Here's how you can prepare this traditional delight at home:

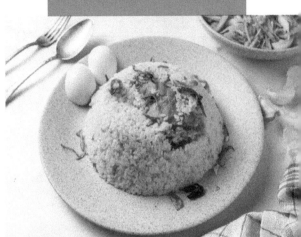

Ingredients:

For the Chicken (Morog) Marination:
- **1** kg chicken, cut into medium-sized pieces
- **1** cup yogurt
- **2** tablespoons ginger-garlic paste
- **2** teaspoons turmeric powder
- **2** teaspoons red chili powder (adjust to taste)
- **1** teaspoon garam masala
- Salt to taste
- **2** tablespoons mustard oil (or any cooking oil)

For the Rice (Polao):
- **2** cups Basmati rice (or any long-grain rice)
- **4** cups water
- **2** onions, thinly sliced
- **2** bay leaves
- **4-5** green cardamom pods
- **4-5** cloves
- **1**-inch cinnamon stick
- **2** tablespoons ghee or clarified butter
- Salt to taste

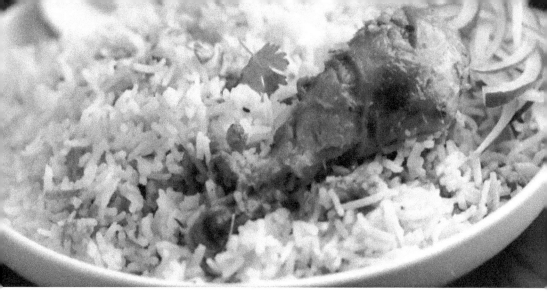

Instructions:

1. Marinate the Chicken: Mix the chicken pieces with yogurt, ginger-garlic paste, turmeric powder, red chili powder, garam masala, salt, and mustard oil. Let it marinate for at least 2 hours or overnight for best results.

2. Prepare the Rice: Wash the rice grains under running water until the water runs clear. Soak them in water for 30 minutes. Drain.

3. In a large pot or deep pan, heat ghee or clarified butter. Add the sliced onions and fry until they become golden brown. Remove half of the fried onions and set aside for garnishing later.

4. To the same pot, add the bay leaves, cardamom, cloves, and cinnamon stick. Fry for a minute or until aromatic.

5. Add the marinated chicken to the pot and fry on high heat for 5-6 minutes until the chicken gets a nice sear on the outside.

6. Lower the heat and cook the chicken for another 10-12 minutes, occasionally stirring.

7. Now, add the drained rice to the pot and gently mix. Add 4 cups of water and salt. Stir carefully to ensure the rice and chicken are well combined.

8. Bring the mixture to a boil. Once most of the water has evaporated and the rice starts to show on the surface, reduce the heat to the lowest setting, cover the pot with a tight-fitting lid, and let it simmer for 20-25 minutes.

9. Once done, turn off the heat and let the Morog Polao sit for another 10 minutes.

10. Before serving, fluff the rice with a fork and garnish with the reserved fried onions. Enjoy the Morog Polao with a side of raita, salad, or just a wedge of lemon. This flavorful dish encapsulates the essence of Dhakai cuisine, making every bite memorable!

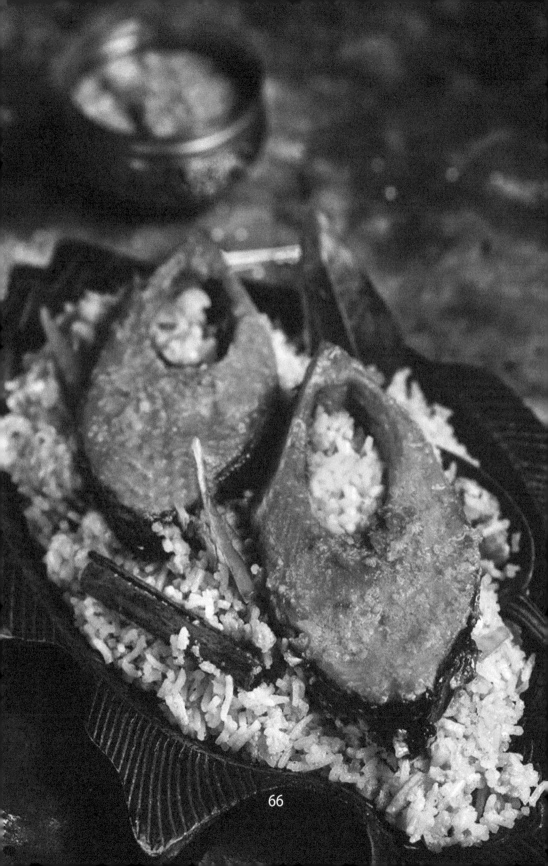

Ilish Biryani

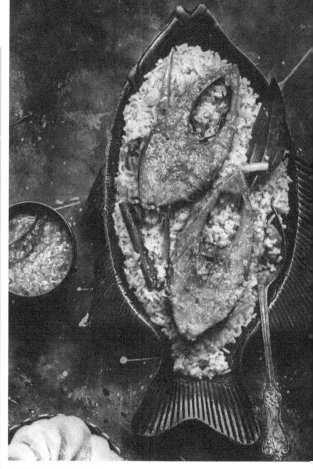

Ilish or Hilsa fish is a delicacy in Bangladesh. It's renowned for its unique taste and is deeply embedded in the culture and traditions of the region. Combining Ilish with Biryani, another beloved dish, creates an exquisite culinary experience. Here's how you can prepare Ilish Biryani:

Ingredients:

For the Ilish Marination:
- 6 pieces of Ilish (Hilsa) fish, cleaned and sliced
- 1 tablespoon turmeric powder
- 2 teaspoons red chili powder
- Salt to taste
- Juice of 1 le mon

For the Rice:
- **2** cups Basmati rice
- **4** cups water
- 2 bay leaves
- **4-5** green cardamom pods
- **4-5** cloves
- **1**-inch cinnamon stick
- Salt to taste

For the Biryani Gravy:
- **2** onions, thinly sliced
- **1** tomato, finely chopped
- **2** tablespoons ginger-garlic paste
- **2** green chilies, slit
- **1/2** cup yogurt
- **2** teaspoons Biryani masala or garam masala
- A handful of fresh coriander leaves, chopped
- A handful of fresh mint leaves, chopped
- **3** tablespoons mustard oil (or any other cooking oil)
- Salt to taste

67

Instructions:

1. **Marinate the Ilish:** Rub the Ilish pieces with turmeric, red chili powder, salt, and lemon juice. Allow them to marinate for at least 30 minutes.

2. **Prepare the Rice:** Wash the rice several times until the water is clear. Soak for about 30 minutes, then drain. In a large pot, boil water with bay leaves, cardamom, cloves, cinnamon, and salt. Add the rice and cook until it's 70% done. Drain the water and spread the rice on a tray to cool.

3. **Cooking the Ilish:** In a pan, heat mustard oil. Once hot, gently place the marinated Ilish pieces and fry for 1-2 minutes on each side, ensuring they don't break. Remove and set aside.

4. In the same oil, add sliced onions. Fry until they turn golden brown. Add the ginger-garlic paste and green chilies, and sauté for 2 minutes. Introduce the chopped tomato and cook until it becomes soft.

5. Lower the heat and add yogurt, biryani masala, salt, half of the chopped mint, and coriander leaves.
Mix well.

6. Gently place the fried Ilish pieces into this gravy. Allow them to simmer for about 5 minutes.

7. **Layering the Biryani:** In a large pot, layer the partially cooked rice over the Ilish and its gravy. Sprinkle the remaining mint and coriander leaves on top.

8. Cover the pot with a tight-fitting lid. You can also seal it using dough or use a heavy pan on top to ensure no steam escapes.

9. Cook on very low heat for about 25-30 minutes. This process allows all the flavors to meld.

10. **Serve:** Carefully open the pot and serve the Ilish Biryani hot with your choice of raita or salad. This Ilish Biryani, with its rich flavors and aromatic rice, is a testament to the brilliance of Bangladeshi cuisine. Enjoy!

Section 5.5:
The Art of Cooking Biryani

Biryani is not just a dish; it's a symphony of aromas, flavors, and textures that come together in a sublime culinary creation. The very essence of biryani lies in its meticulous preparation and layers of ingredients that perfectly harmonize with each other.

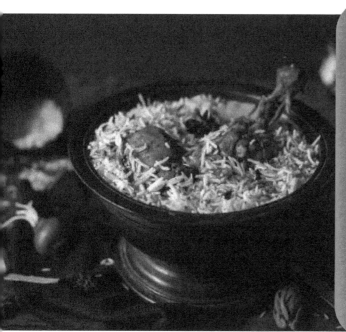

The Origin: While biryani's roots can be traced back to various regions of the Indian subcontinent, the Bangladeshi variant has carved out its own niche. Here, it's often infused with local spices, freshwater fish or succulent meat, making it distinctively flavorful.

The Spices: Every biryani's soul is its blend of spices. From the fragrant cardamom to the pungent star anise, each spice has a role to play. The Bangladeshi version often includes keora water (screw pine essence) and sometimes rose water, giving it a unique aromatic signature.

The Rice: A good biryani demands long-grained rice, usually the Basmati variety, that remains separate yet fully absorbs the flavors of the spices. The rice should be partially cooked separately before layering, ensuring it doesn't turn mushy during the 'dum' process.

The Accolades: There's a reason why biryani is often the centerpiece at Bangladeshi festivities. Its tantalizing aroma draws you in, and the delectable taste ensures it's remembered long after the meal ends. Families often have their guarded biryani recipes, passed down generations, each boasting its distinct flavor profile.

Pairings: A well-made biryani doesn't need much by its side, but raita (a yogurt-based side dish), a tangy brinjal (eggplant) preparation, or a simple salad can complement it.

As we further delve into the world of Bangladeshi cuisine in subsequent sections, we'll uncover lighter,
more refreshing elements that contrast and complement the rich, profound nature of biryani. Await a voyage into crisp salads, zesty chutneys, and other delightful accompaniments that complete the Bangladeshi dining experience.

Section 5.5: The Science Behind the Art of Cooking Biryani

Biryani, a beloved dish in many parts of the world, is as much about art as it is about science. Let's delve into some scientific facts that contribute to the making of this flavorful dish:

1.Maillard Reaction:
The unique flavor and brown color of the meat in biryani come from the Maillard Reaction. When you fry or sear the meat, the amino acids in it react with the sugars at high temperatures, leading to complex flavor compounds. This reaction is responsible for the rich, savory notes in the meat.

2. Rice Starch Gelatinization:
When you cook rice in biryani, the heat causes the starch granules in the rice to swell and absorb water. This process, known as gelatinization, is crucial for getting the right texture in biryani rice. The distinct grains of rice, each separate from the other, are a hallmark of a well-cooked biryani.

3. Steaming (Dum) Technique:
Biryani often employs the 'dum' method - sealing the pot with dough and allowing the biryani to steam in its juices. This method ensures uniform heat distribution, allowing flavors to meld while ensuring that the meat and rice are perfectly cooked. The moisture trapped inside helps in cooking and infusing flavors deeply.

4. Spices Release Essential Oils:
The myriad spices used in biryani release essential oils when heated, which are volatile compounds responsible for their characteristic flavors and aromas. The layering technique in biryani ensures that these flavors are evenly distributed throughout the dish.

5. Acidic Ingredients:
Ingredients like yogurt or tomatoes, which are often used in biryani marinades, are acidic. This acidity can help in tenderizing the meat. The proteins in the meat break down in acidic conditions, making it softer and allowing it to absorb more flavors.

6. Saffron's Color Diffusion:
The vibrant yellow or orange streaks in biryani come from saffron soaked in milk or water. The warm liquid helps extract the color from the saffron threads, which is a result of the diffusion of crocin, a natural carotenoid chemical responsible for saffron's hue.

These scientific principles, combined with the chef's expertise and intuition, make biryani a dish that's both flavorful and texturally perfect. It's a beautiful blend of tradition, art, and science.

Fish

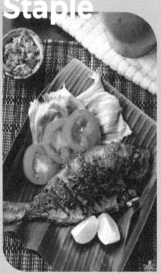

Chapter 6: Fish - The Bangladeshi Staple

Fish, with its rich nutritional profile and versatile culinary applications, is a central part of Bangladeshi cuisine. Given the country's abundant freshwater resources, a plethora of fish species find their way into local dishes. This chapter uncovers a range of authentic, traditional fish recipes that have been passed down through generations.

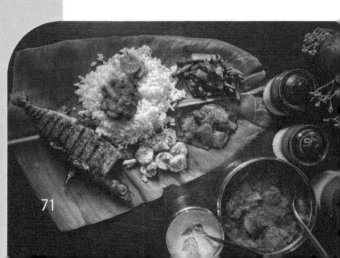

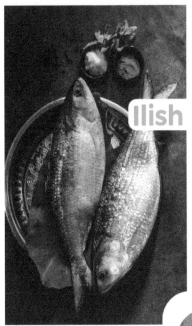

Section 6.1:
Ilish - The Queen of Fish

We cannot talk about Bangladeshi fish recipes without mentioning the beloved Hilsa, or Ilish, fish. 'Ilish Bhapa', a dish where the fish is marinated in mustard sauce and steamed to perfection, and 'Ilish Polao', a rich rice dish cooked with Hilsa, are among the many ways this fish is savored.

Ilish Bhapa Recipe

Ingredients:
- 500g ....Hilsa fish
- 2 ....tablespoons mustard seeds
- 2 ....green chillies
- 1/2 ....teaspoon turmeric powder
- ....Salt to taste
- ....Mustard oil for drizzling

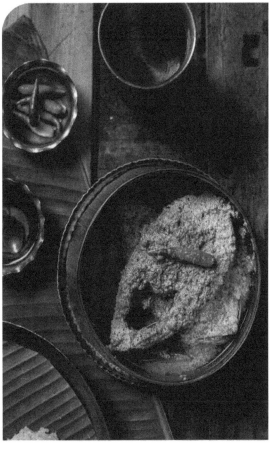

Instructions:
1. Soak the mustard seeds in a little bit o water for 10-15 minutes.
2. In a blender, add the soaked mustarc seeds, green chillies, turmeric, and salt Blend to make a smooth paste.
3. Marinate the Hilsa fish with the preparec mustard paste and let it rest for 30 minutes
4. Place the fish on a steaming tray, drizzle with mustard oil, and steam for about 10-15 minutes or until the fish is cooked through.
5. Serve the Ilish Bhapa hot with a side of steamed rice.

Section 6.2: Rui and Katla - The Everyday Fish

'Rui' (Rohu) and 'Katla' are common choices for everyday cooking. They are used in various dishes such as 'Doi Maach' (fish in yogurt gravy), 'Maacher Jhol' (fish in a light, spicy broth), and 'Maacher Kalia' (a rich, spicy fish curry).

Doi Maach Recipe

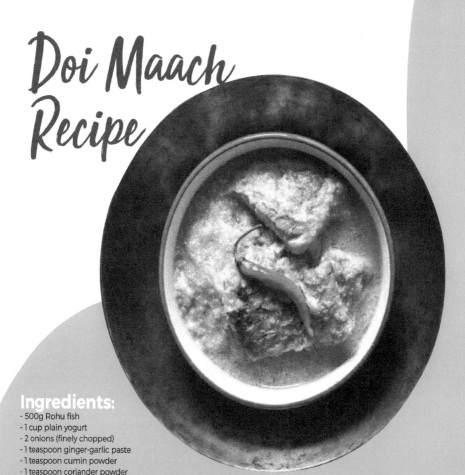

Ingredients:
- 500g Rohu fish
- 1 cup plain yogurt
- 2 onions (finely chopped)
- 1 teaspoon ginger-garlic paste
- 1 teaspoon cumin powder
- 1 teaspoon coriander powder
- 1/2 teaspoon turmeric powder
- Salt to taste
- Vegetable oil for frying

Instructions:

1. Marinate the Rohu fish with salt and turmeric. Let it rest for 15 minutes.

2. Heat oil in a pan and fry the fish until golden brown. Remove from the pan and set aside.

3. In the same pan, add the onions and sauté until golden brown.

4. Add the ginger-garlic paste, cumin powder, coriander powder, and turmeric to the onions. Cook for a few minutes until the spices are well combined.

5. Lower the heat and add the yogurt to the pan. Stir well and cook for a few minutes until the yogurt is well incorporated into the mixture.

6. Add the fried fish to the pan and coat with the yogurt mixture. Cover the pan and cook on low heat for 10-15 minutes.

7. Serve the Doi Maach hot with rice.

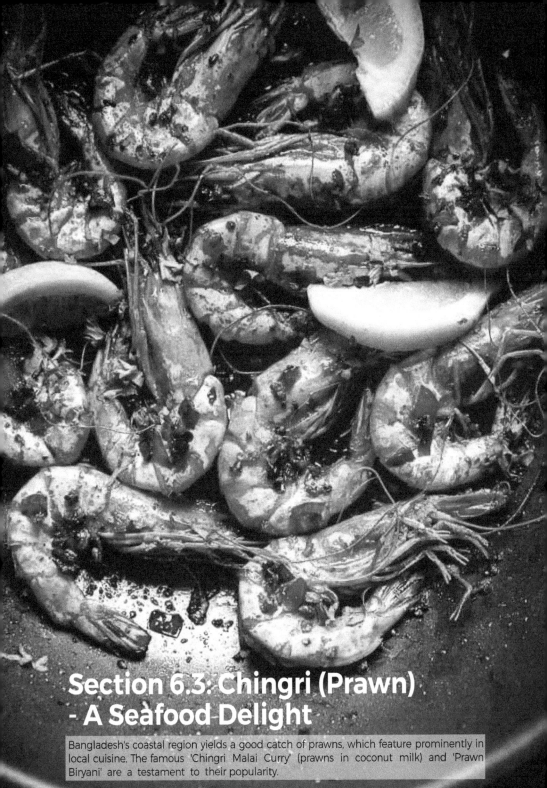

Section 6.3: Chingri (Prawn) - A Seafood Delight

Bangladesh's coastal region yields a good catch of prawns, which feature prominently in local cuisine. The famous 'Chingri Malai Curry' (prawns in coconut milk) and 'Prawn Biryani' are a testament to their popularity.

Chingri Malai Curry

Recipe

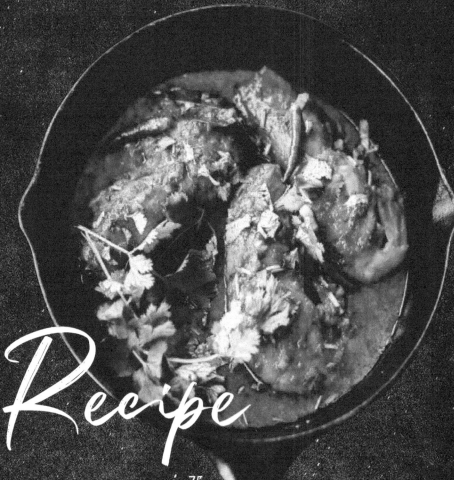

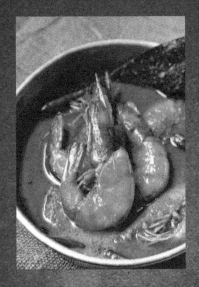

Ingredients:

- 500g   prawns
- 1   can coconut milk
- 2   onions (finely chopped)
- 1   teaspoon ginger paste
- 1   teaspoon garlic paste
- 1/2   teaspoon turmeric powder
-             Salt to taste
-             Vegetable oil for frying

Instructions:

1. Marinate the prawns with salt and turmeric. Let it rest for 15 minutes.
2. Heat oil in a pan and fry the prawns until they turn pink. Remove from the pan and set aside.
3. In the same pan, add the onions and sauté until golden brown.
4. Add the ginger paste and garlic paste to the onions. Cook for a few minutes until the raw smell of the paste disappears.
5. Add the coconut milk, turmeric, and salt to the pan. Stir well and bring to a boil.
6. Add the fried prawns to the pan and cook for a few minutes until the prawns are well coated with the curry.

Please note that the traditional fish bhorta and Paturi recipes are relatively complex, so it's recommended to follow specific recipes from a reliable source to ensure that the dishes are prepared correctly. Enjoy your cooking!

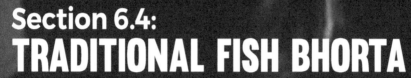

Section 6.4:
TRADITIONAL FISH BHORTA

Fish bhortas, like 'Shutki Bhorta' (dried fish mash), offer an intensely flavourful experience. These are usually served as a side dish with rice and lend a distinct taste to meals.

Traditional Fish Bhorta

Bhorta is a traditional Bangladeshi dish, typically made by mashing boiled or roasted vegetables or fish with mustard oil, green chili, and various spices. Fish bhorta is a delicious variation, where tender pieces of fish are mashed and mixed with fragrant spices. This dish is both flavorful and spicy and is usually enjoyed with plain rice.

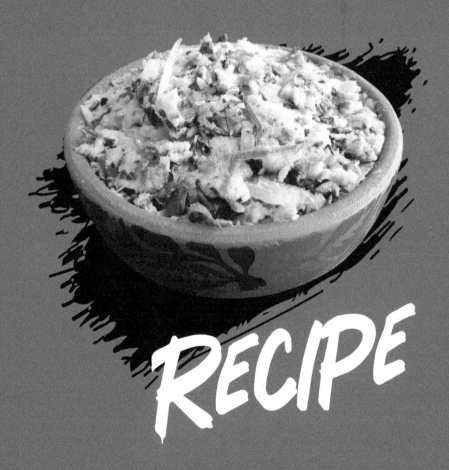

RECIPE

Ingredients:

1. Fish (typically a white-fleshed fish like Hilsa, Rui, or Pangasius) - 250 grams
2. Green chilies - 4 to 5 (or as per taste)
3. Garlic cloves - 3
4. Mustard oil - 3 tablespoons
5. Turmeric powder - 1/2 teaspoon
6. Salt - to taste
7. Fresh coriander leaves - a handful (chopped, for garnish)

Instructions:

1. Preparation of Fish:

a. Clean the fish thoroughly and marinate with turmeric powder and salt.

b. Steam the fish until it is fully cooked. You can also pan-fry or grill the fish if you prefer.

c. Once cooked, remove and discard the bones and skin, leaving only the tender fish flesh.

2. Making the Bhorta:

a. In a large mortar and pestle (or using a grinder), crush the green chilies and garlic cloves into a coarse paste.

b. Add the cooked fish to the mortar and pestle and continue to mash everything together until the mixture becomes relatively smooth. If you don't have a mortar and pestle, you can use a fork to mash the fish and mix it with the chili-garlic paste.

c. Transfer the mixture to a bowl.

3. Seasoning:

a. Drizzle mustard oil over the mashed fish mixture.

b. Add salt to taste and mix everything together until well combined. The mustard oil will give the bhorta its traditional pungent aroma and unique taste.

4. Serving:

a. Transfer the fish bhorta to a serving dish and garnish with chopped fresh coriander leaves.

b. Serve hot with plain steamed rice.

Note: The spiciness of the bhorta can be adjusted by increasing or decreasing the number of green chilies used. This dish is traditionally quite spicy, but it can be tailored to your preference.

Paturi - Fish in Banana Leaf Recipe

Paturi is a traditional culinary delight from Bangladesh where fish is marinated with spices and then wrapped in a banana leaf before being steamed or grilled. This cooking process not only keeps the fish moist but also infuses it with the delicate aroma of the banana leaf. Most commonly, Hilsa fish (Ilish) is used for this dish, but other fish can be substituted based on availability.

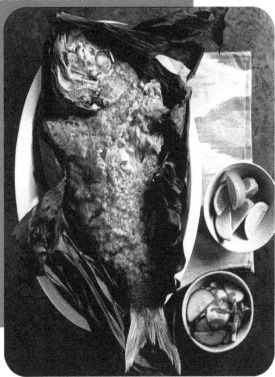

Ingredients:

1. Fish steaks or fillets - **4** pieces (preferably Hilsa, but you can use any white-fleshed fish)
2. Banana leaves - **4** (large enough to wrap each fish piece)
3. Mustard seeds - **2** tablespoons
4. Green chilies - **5-6** (or to taste)
5. Turmeric powder - **1** teaspoon
6. Yogurt - **2** tablespoons
7. Mustard oil - **3** tablespoons
8. Salt - to taste
9. Cotton string or toothpicks to secure the banana leaf parcels

Instructions:

1. Marinate the Fish:

A. In a blender, combine mustard seeds, green chilies, turmeric powder, yogurt, and salt. Blend into a smooth paste.

B. Place the fish pieces in a bowl and pour over the mustard paste. Ensure each piece is well-coated with the marinade.

C. Drizzle mustard oil over the fish, mix gently, and let it marinate for at least 30 minutes.

2. Prepare the Banana Leaves:

A. Soften the banana leaves by quickly passing them over an open flame. This makes them pliable and prevents tearing.

B. Cut the leaves into squares or rectangles, large enough to wrap around the fish pieces.

3. Wrapping and Cooking:

A. Place a fish piece in the center of a banana leaf square. Pour a spoonful of the marinade over the fish.

B. Fold the banana leaf over the fish, forming a parcel. Secure the parcel with a cotton string or toothpick.

C. Repeat this process for all the fish pieces.

D. Steam the fish parcels for about **15-20** minutes, ensuring they are fully cooked and infused with the flavors from the marinade and banana leaf. Alternatively, you can grill them on a barbecue for a smoky flavor.

4. Serving:

A. Serve the Paturi hot, allowing guests to unwrap their own banana leaf parcel, revealing the flavorful and aromatic fish inside.

B. It pairs well with plain steamed rice or pulao.

Culinary Note: The charm of Paturi lies in its simple, yet rich flavors. The banana leaf not only adds to the aesthetic appeal of the dish but also contributes a subtle earthy aroma that elevates the overall taste. Paturi exemplifies the brilliance of Bangladeshi cuisine, where fresh ingredients combined with traditional methods create culinary masterpieces.

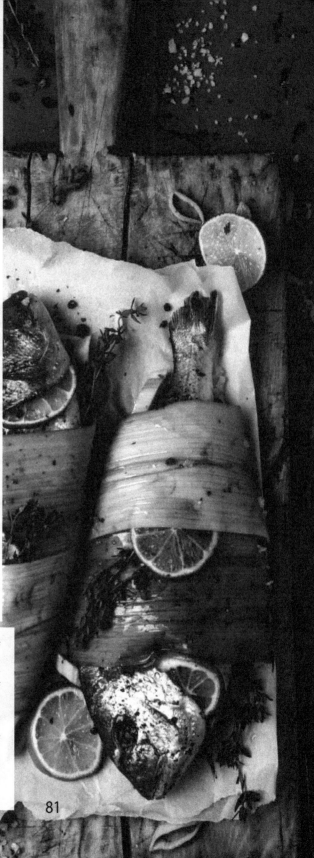

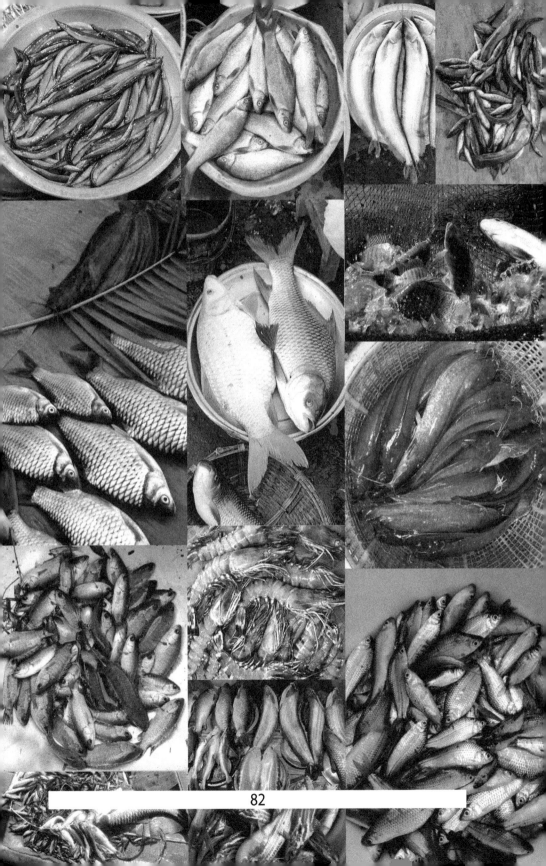

BANGLADESHI FISH CHARACTERISTICS

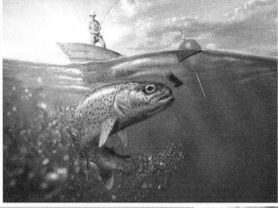

Bangladesh, with its extensive network of rivers, deltas, and the Bay of Bengal, is renowned for its diverse fish fauna. Fish is an integral part of Bangladeshi cuisine and culture. Here are some characteristics of Bangladeshi fish:

1. Diverse Species:

Bangladesh boasts over 260 freshwater fish species. Common varieties include Rohu, Katla, Mrigel, and various types of carp. There are also numerous marine fish species found in the Bay of Bengal, including Hilsa, the national fish of Bangladesh.

2. Anadromous Fish:

Hilsa (or Ilish) is an anadromous fish, meaning it migrates from the sea to freshwater rivers to spawn. The journey of Hilsa and its cultural significance, especially during the monsoon season, is deeply embedded in Bangladeshi culture.

3. Adaptations to Muddy Waters:

Many fish in Bangladesh have adapted to the muddy, turbid waters of its rivers. These adaptations might include a highly developed lateral line (a system of tactile sense organs located in the head and along both sides of the body) or downturned mouths that help in bottom-feeding.

4. Seasonal Variations:

Due to the monsoonal climate, fish availability and breeding patterns often exhibit seasonal variations. Some species spawn during the monsoon season when the water levels rise.

5. Small Indigenous Species (SIS):

Apart from the major carp species, there are many small indigenous fish species in Bangladesh. They are nutritionally rich and an essential part of the rural diet. Examples include mola, chela, and punti.

6. Threats and Conservation:

Many fish species in Bangladesh are under threat due to overfishing, pollution, habitat destruction, and the impacts of climate change, especially rising sea levels and increasing salinity in water. Conservation efforts are underway, but they often compete with the needs and habits of the local population.

7. Cultural Significance:

Fish not only holds dietary significance in Bangladesh but also cultural. Fish motifs are common in art, literature, and daily life. The Bengali proverb "Mach-e Bhat-e Bangali" (Fish and rice make a Bengali) underscores this sentiment.

8. Economic Importance:

Fishing is a significant source of livelihood for millions in Bangladesh. The Sundarbans, the world's largest mangrove forest situated in Bangladesh, acts as a breeding ground for numerous marine and freshwater fish species, supporting the local fisheries sector.

In summary, the fish of Bangladesh are as diverse and dynamic as the country's landscapes and waterways. They hold immense ecological, cultural, and economic value, making their conservation and sustainable use paramount.

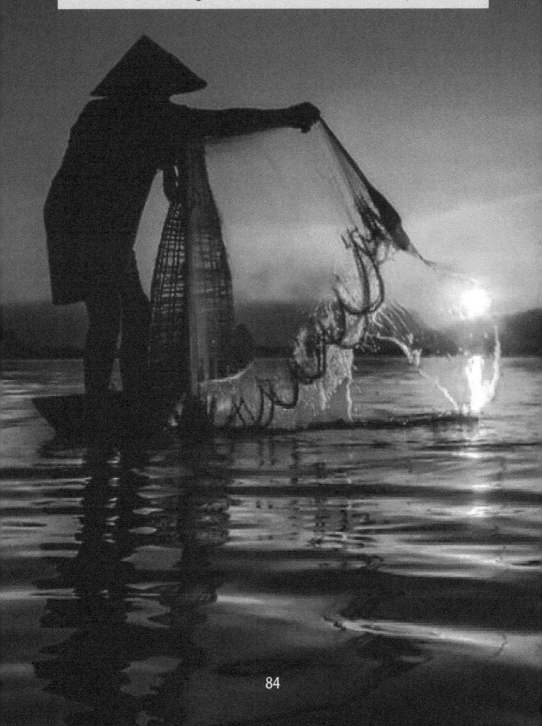

Section 6.7: **Why fish spoils so fast**

Fish spoil rapidly due to a combination of their biological makeup and the bacteria that thrive in aquatic environments. Here are the primary reasons why fish spoil faster than many other meats:

1. High Enzymatic Activity:
Fish muscles contain enzymes that, once the fish is caught and dies, begin to break down its tissues. This enzymatic action can lead to softening of the flesh and changes in flavor, which are characteristic signs of spoilage.

2. Neutral pH:
The flesh of most fish has a neutral pH, which provides an ideal environment for bacteria to grow. Some of these bacteria can produce compounds that have off-flavors or are spoilage indicators.

3. Presence of Bacteria:
The aquatic environment is rich in microorganisms. When fish are caught, their skin, gills, and intestines often carry a load of these bacteria, including spoilage bacteria and pathogens. Once the fish is dead and its immune system is no longer active, these bacteria proliferate, leading to rapid spoilage.

4. High Moisture Content:
Fish flesh has a high water content, which provides an ideal medium for bacterial growth. Bacteria thrive in moist environments, which accelerates the spoilage process.

7. Temperature Sensitivity:
Fish are cold-blooded animals, which means they don't regulate their body temperature like mammals do. As a result, their bodies are usually at the same temperature as the water they live in. When fish are caught from cold waters and then exposed to warmer temperatures, their tissues can deteriorate rapidly.

6. High Protein Content:
The high protein content in fish makes it a rich source of nutrients not just for humans but also for bacteria. As bacteria break down these proteins, they produce compounds like amines and sulfur, which contribute to the foul smell associated with spoiled fish.

5. Unsaturated Fatty Acids:
Many fish, especially those termed as "fatty fish" like salmon, mackerel, and sardines, have high levels of unsaturated fatty acids. While these fatty acids are beneficial for human health, they oxidize quickly when exposed to air. This oxidation leads to the development of rancid flavors and off-odors.

To combat the rapid spoilage of fish:

- It's crucial to store fish at cold temperatures immediately after catching.
- Proper handling, cleaning, and storage can significantly extend the shelf life of fish.
- Consuming fish as soon as possible after purchase or catching is always
  recommended for the best quality and safety.

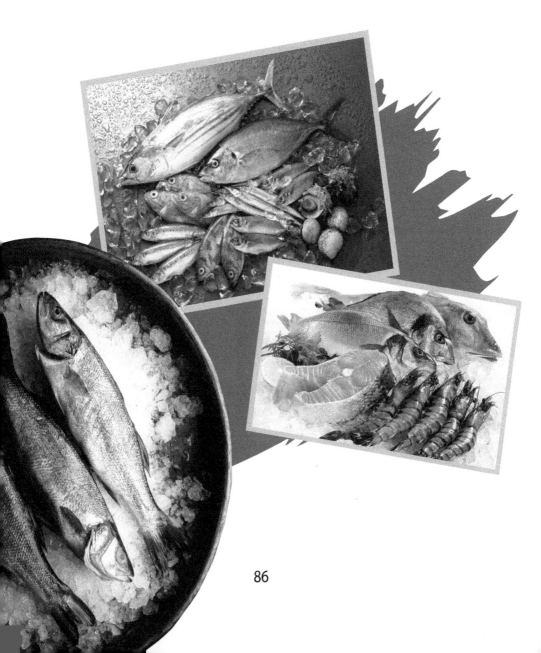

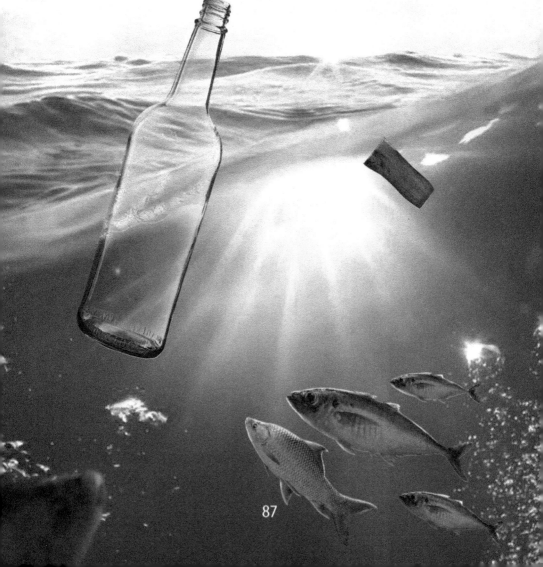

Section 6.8: Bangladeshi Fish Worldwide:
A FRESH BUSINESS IDEA

Introduction:

Bangladesh, with its rich river networks and a coastline along the Bay of Bengal, is home to a diverse range of fish species. Bangladeshi fish is known not only for its diversity but also its unique taste and nutritional benefits. As global food preferences evolve and there's a growing demand for authentic, ethnic cuisines, introducing Bangladeshi fish to a worldwide market offers a lucrative business opportunity.

1. Business Idea - Exporting Authentic Bangladeshi Fish:

Launch an export-oriented business focusing on delivering fresh, frozen, or processed Bangladeshi fish varieties to international markets.

2. Potential Fish Varieties:

- Hilsa (Ilish): The national fish of Bangladesh, known for its delicate flavor and rich, oily texture.
- Rui (Rohu): A popular freshwater fish, vital in Bangladeshi cuisine.
- Katla: Another major freshwater fish that's highly sought after.
- Pangasius: Gaining popularity internationally for its neutral flavor and firm texture.
- Chingri (Prawn): Especially the Bagda and Galda varieties.

3. Value Proposition:

- Authenticity: Provide an authentic taste of Bangladesh to diaspora communities and introduce others to the unique flavors of Bangladeshi fish.
- Health Benefits: Highlight the health benefits of consuming fish, such as omega-3 fatty acids, lean protein, and essential vitamins.

4. Business Model Considerations:

- Supply Chain Management: Ensure a seamless cold chain for fresh and frozen fish export. Collaborate with local fishermen and fisheries to ensure a consistent supply.
- Quality Assurance: Adhere to international standards and certifications to ensure the quality, safety, and sustainability of fishery practices.
- Branding: Create a brand that resonates with both authenticity and quality. Use storytelling to communicate the cultural significance and flavors of Bangladeshi fish.
- Market Research: Understand the preferences of the target markets. Diaspora communities could be the initial focus, expanding later to other demographics.
- Local Partnerships: Collaborate with restaurants and stores in target countries to promote Bangladeshi fish through special dishes or promotional events.

5. Challenges:

- Regulatory Compliance: Navigating export-import regulations and ensuring compliance with food safety standards in target countries.
- Sustainability: Ensuring sustainable fishing practices to protect both the environment and the long-term viability of the business.
- Logistics: Managing the logistics of transporting perishable goods internationally.

6. Monetization:

- Direct Sales: Export to international markets for sale in supermarkets, ethnic grocery stores, or specialized seafood outlets.
- Partnerships: Collaborate with restaurants worldwide, introducing Bangladeshi fish specials.
- Online Marketplace: Launch an online platform selling fresh or frozen fish directly to consumers.

Conclusion:

Exporting Bangladeshi fish worldwide capitalizes on the growing demand for authentic, ethnic food products. By ensuring quality, sustainability, and effective branding, this business idea holds potential to not only capture the tastes of Bangladeshi diaspora but also introduce the unique flavors of Bangladeshi fish to global consumers. With careful planning and execution, this venture can contribute to global culinary diversity while generating significant economic benefits.

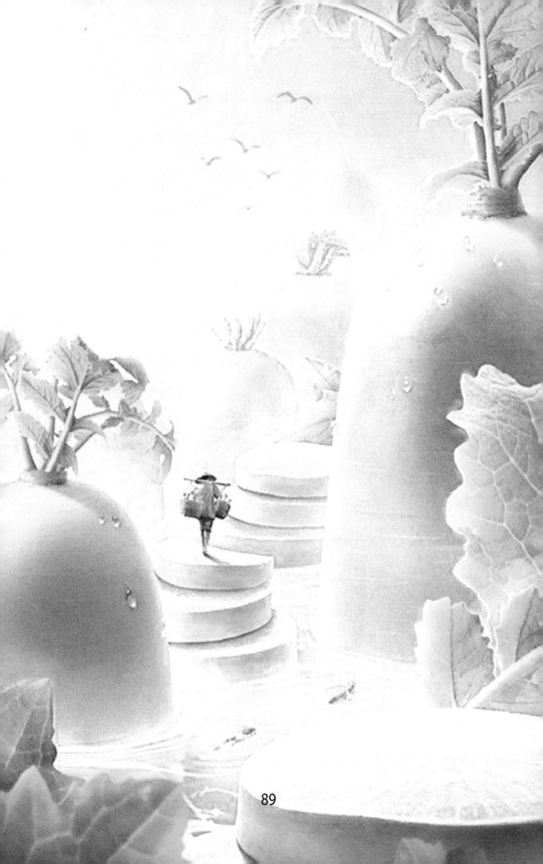

Chapter 7: Bangladeshi Vegetarian and Vegan Delight

Bangladesh, with its fertile lands and favorable climate, is abundant in fresh fruits, vegetables, and legumes, providing ample ingredients for a vibrant vegetarian and vegan cuisine. This chapter delves into the world of plant-based Bangladeshi cooking, showcasing recipes that are flavorful, rich, and diverse.

Section 7.1: Daal - The Everyday Essential

'Cholar Daal' (split chickpeas), 'Masoor Daal' (red lentils), and 'Moog Daal ' (mung beans) are central to Bangladeshi cuisine. Prepared with various spices, these lentil dishes form an integral part of every meal, providing essential proteins.

Masoor Daal

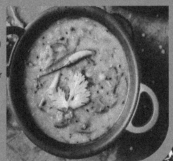

Ingredients:
- 1 cup red lentils (Masoor Daal)
- 1 onion, chopped
- 2 green chilies, sliced
- 1/2 teaspoon turmeric powder
- Salt to taste
- 2 tablespoons oil
- 1 teaspoon cumin seeds
- 3 cloves garlic, minced

Instructions:
1. Rinse the lentils thoroughly and add them to a pot with 3 cups of water, the chopped onion, gree n chilies, turmeric, and salt.
2. Bring the mixture to a boil, then reduce the heat and simmer until the lentils are soft and the consistency is somewhat creamy.
3. In a separate pan, heat the oil and add the cumin seeds. Once they start to crackle, add th e minced garlic and sauté until golden brown.
4. Pour this garlic and cumin 'tarka' over the cooked lentils and stir well.
5. Serve the Masoor Daal with rice or roti.

Bangladesh's coastal region yields a good catch of prawns, which feature prominently in local cuisine. The famous 'Chingri Malai Curry' (prawns in coconut milk) and 'Prawn Biryani' are a testament to their popularity.

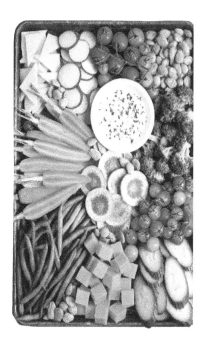

Section 7.2: **Shobji - The Versatile Vegetable** *Dishes*

Vegetable dishes, or 'Shobji', play a significant role in Bangladeshi meals, providing nutrition and balance. They can be enjoyed as main dishes or as accompaniments. Below are a few classic recipes that showcase the variety and depth of flavors in 'Shobji'.

1. Begun Bhaja
(Fried Eggplant Slices)

Ingredients:

- Eggplant - 1 large, cut into round slices
- Turmeric powder - 1 tsp
- Red chili powder - 1/2 tsp (optional)
- Salt - to taste
- Mustard oil - for frying

Instructions:

1. Sprinkle the eggplant slices with salt, turmeric, and red chili powder. Mix well to ensure each slice is coated evenly.
2. Heat mustard oil in a pan until it's hot but not smoking.
3. Place the eggplant slices in the pan and fry each side until it's golden brown and crispy.
4. Remove from oil and drain on paper towels. Serve hot.

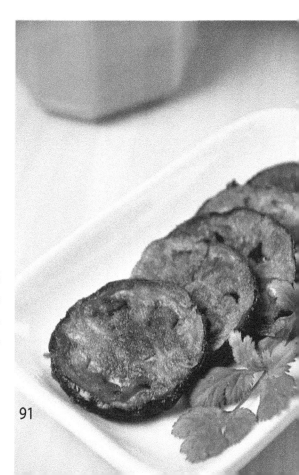

Alu Bhorta (Mashed Potatoes)

Ingredients:

- 4 potatoes
- 1 onion, finely chopped
- 2 green chilies, finely chopped
- Salt to taste
- 2 tbsp mustard oil

Instructions:

1. Boil the potatoes until soft.

2. Peel the potatoes and mash them.

3. Add the chopped onions, chilies, salt, and mustard oil. Mix well.

4. Serve with rice.

3. LAU GHONTO

(Bottle Gourd Curry)

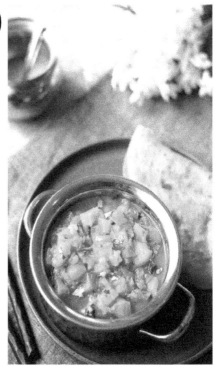

Ingredients:

- Bottle gourd (Lau) - 1 medium-sized, peeled and diced
- Panch phoron (Bengali five-spice blend) - 1 tsp
- Green chilies - 2, slit
- Turmeric powder - 1 tsp
- Salt - to taste
- Mustard oil - 2 tbsp
- Warm water - 1 cup

Instructions:

1. Heat mustard oil in a pan and add the panch phoron. Once it startsto splutter, add the slit green chilies.
2. Add the diced bottle gourd, followed by turmeric and salt. Mix well.
3. Pour in the warm water, cover the pan with a lid, and let it simmer until the bottle gourd is cooked and tender.
4. Check for seasoning and adjust if necessary. Once done, remove from heat.

Culinary Note: While these dishes are quite simple, they hold an esteemed place in Bangladeshi cuisine. 'Shobji' dishes reflect the importance of fresh ingredients and the beauty of minimalist cooking, where each ingredient shines through, complmenting the others. These recipes can be enjoyed with rice or flatbreads and offer a satisfying, comforting, and healthful eating experience.

The Dairy and Non-Dairy Alternatives

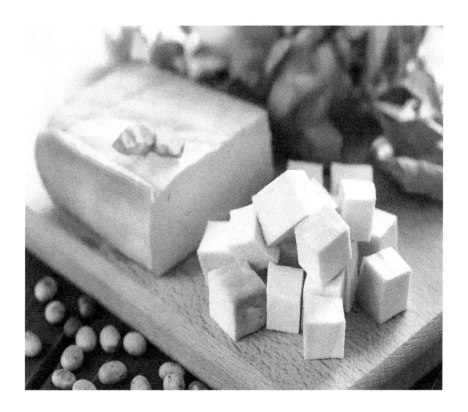

Though not traditionally used in Bangladeshi cuisine, Paneer (cottage cheese) and Tofu are gaining popularity in contemporary cooking. Paneer Jalfrezi and Tofu Bhuna are tasty dishes, rich in protein and compatible with a vegetarian or vegan diet.

HOW TO MAKE PANEER
(Cottage Cheese)

Ingredients:

1. 1 liter whole milk
2. 2-3 tablespoons lemon juice or white vinegar
   (you can also use yogurt or citric acid)

Instructions:

1. Boil Milk: Pour the milk into a heavy-bottomed pan and bring it to a boil. Keep stirring occasionally to ensure that the milk does not stick to the bottom of the pan.

2. Add Acid: Once the milk has come to a boil, turn off the heat. Add the lemon juice or vinegar a little at a time, stirring the milk gently. You'll see the milk curdling.

3. Separate Curds and Whey: Once the milk is fully curdled, you'll notice greenish whey separated from the milk solids.

4. Strain: Place a muslin cloth or cheesecloth over a strainer. Pour the curdled milk through the cloth to separate the curds from the whey. You can save the whey; it's nutritious and can be used in breads, soups, or curries.

5. Set the Paneer: Rinse the curds under cold water to get rid of the lemony/vinegar taste. Gather the cloth's corners and twist to squeeze out more liquid. Now, shape the paneer into a block, still wrapped in the cloth. Place a heavy object on top to help set the paneer and remove all the water. Leave it for a few hours.

6. Unwrap and Store: Once set, unwrap the paneer. It's now ready to be used in your dishes! If you're not using it immediately, store it in the refrigerator. It's best used within 3-4 days.

HOW TO MAKE TOFU
(Bean Curd)

Ingredients:

1. 2 cups dried soybeans
2. 2 teaspoons liquid nigari or calcium sulfate (gypsum) as a coagulant

1. Soak the Soybeans:

Soak the dried soybeans overnight in plenty of water. They will expand quite a bit.

2. Blend:

Drain and rinse the soybeans. In a blender, blend the soaked beans with fresh water (about 3 cups). Blend until it's smooth.

3. Boil the Soybean Mixture:

Pour the mixture into a large pot and add another 3 cups of water. Bring this to a boil while stirring occasionally. Reduce the heat and let it simmer for about 10 minutes.

4. Strain:

Use a muslin or cheesecloth to strain the mixture into a large bowl. The liquid is soy milk, and the residue left behind is called okara, which can be used in other recipes.

5. Coagulate:

Bring the soy milk to a boil again and then let it cool to about 70 -80°C. Add the coagulant (nigari or calcium sulfate) dissolved in some warm water. Stir gently and then let it sit f or 15-20 minutes. The soy milk will curdle and become tofu.

6. Press:

Pour the curdled soy milk into a mold lined with a cheesecloth. Place a weight on top and let it sit for at least 30 minutes to several hours, depending on the desired firmness.

7. Unmold and Store:

Unwrap the tofu from the cloth and immerse it in cold water. It can be stored in the refrigerator, submerged in water, for up to a week. Make sure to change the water every day. Both paneer and tofu are versatile ingredients and can be used in a variety of recipes. They are a great source of protein, especially for those following a vegetarian or vegan diet.

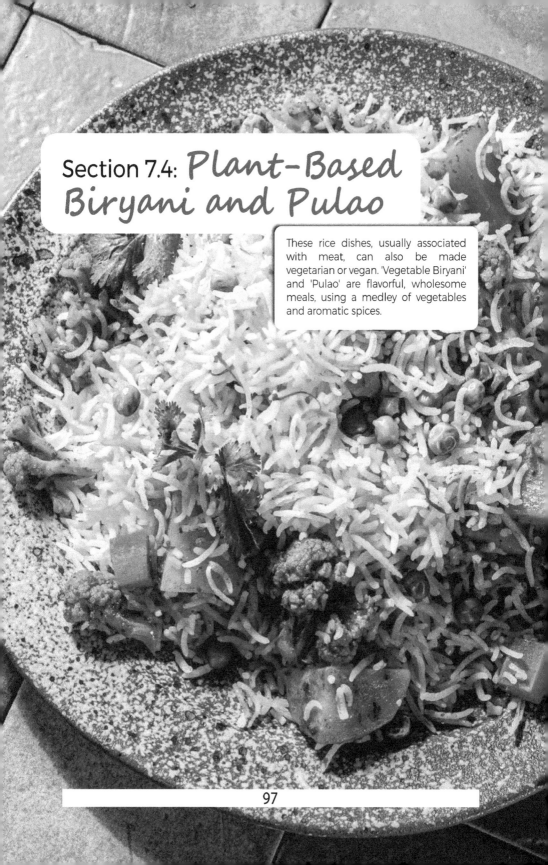

Section 7.4: Plant-Based Biryani and Pulao

These rice dishes, usually associated with meat, can also be made vegetarian or vegan. 'Vegetable Biryani' and 'Pulao' are flavorful, wholesome meals, using a medley of vegetables and aromatic spices.

Vegetable Biryani Recipe

Ingredients:

cups Basmati rice	- 2
onion, thinly sliced	- 1
carrot, diced	- 1
bell pepper, diced	- 1
cup cauliflower florets	- 1
tablespoons vegetable oil	- 2
teaspoons Biryani spice mix	- 2
Salt to taste	-

Instructions:

1. Rinse the rice thoroughly until the water runs clear. Soak the rice in water for 30 minutes, then drain.
2. In a large pan, heat the oil and add the sliced onion. Sauté until golden brown.
3. Add the diced carrot, bell pepper, and cauliflower to the pan and cook for a few minutes until the vegetables are slightly tender.
4. Add the Biryani spice mix and salt to the pan and stir well to coat the vegetables.
5. Add the drained rice to the pan and stir gently to mix with the vegetables and spices.
6. Add 4 cups of water to the pan and bring to a boil. Reduce the heat to low, cover the pan, and cook until the rice is tender and the water has been absorbed.
7. Serve the Vegetable Biryani hot with a side of raita or salad.

Paneer and Tofu

The Dairy and Non-Dairy Alternatives

As global culinary influences mingle with traditional practices, ingredients like paneer and tofu find a place in the hearts and kitchens of Bangladesh. *Their versatility* and protein-rich content make them favorites among both vegetarians and non-vegetarians. Here are two delightful recipes that incorporate these ingredients into Bangladeshi flavors:

1. Paneer Jalfrezi

Ingredients:
- Paneer - 250 grams, cut into strips or cubes
- Bell peppers (red, green, and yellow) - 1 each, thinly sliced
- Onion - 1 large, thinly sliced
- Tomato - 2, finely chopped
- Ginger-garlic paste - 1 tsp
- Turmeric powder - 1/2 tsp
- Red chili powder - 1 tsp
- Garam masala - 1/2 tsp
- Cumin seeds - 1/2 tsp
- Mustard oil or vegetable oil - 2 tbsp
- Salt - to taste
- Fresh coriander - for garnish

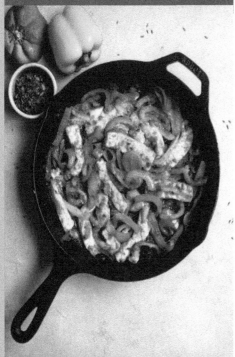

Instructions:

1. Heat oil in a pan and add cumin seeds.

2. Once they splutter, add the sliced onions and sauté until translucent.

3. Add the ginger-garlic paste and sauté for another minute.

4. Mix in the chopped tomatoes and cook until they are soft.

5. Add turmeric powder, red chili powder, and salt. Mix well.

6. Introduce the paneer strips or cubes and the sliced bell peppers.

7. Cook for a few minutes, ensuring the paneer remains soft.

8. Finish with garam masala and garnish with fresh coriander. Serve hot.

2. Tofu Bhuna

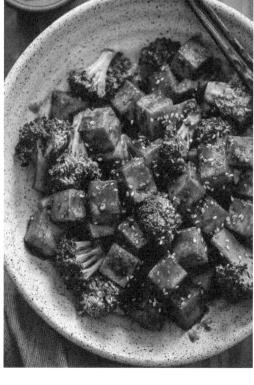

Ingredients:

- Tofu - 250 grams, pressed and cut into cubes
- Onion - 1 large, finely chopped
- Tomato - 2, pureed
- Ginger-garlic paste - 1 tsp
- Turmeric powder - 1/2 tsp
- Red chili powder - 1 tsp
- Cumin powder - 1/2 tsp
- Coriander powder - 1 tsp
- Garam masala - 1/2 tsp
- Mustard oil or vegetable oil - 2 tbsp
- Salt - to taste
- Fresh coriander - for garnish

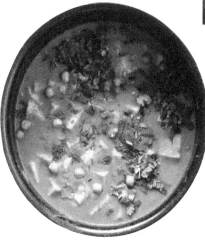

Instructions:

1. In a pan, heat oil and saute onions until golden brown.
2. Add ginger-garlic paste and fry for a minute.
3. Pour in the tomato puree and mix well.
4. Season with turmeric powder, red chili powder, cumin powder, coriander powder, and salt.
5. Once the oil starts to separate from the masala, add the tofu cubes.
6. Gently stir and let the tofu soak up the flavors for 5-7 minutes.
7. Sprinkle garam masala on top and mix gently.
8. Garnish with chopped coriander and serve.

Culinary Note: Both Paneer Jalfrezi and Tofu Bhuna can be paired with naan, paratha, or rice. The robust flavors of these dishes make them perfect for special occasions or when one wants to try something different from regular Bangladeshi fare. Their nutritional value, combined with rich textures and flavors, ensures they're cherished by all.

Enjoy cooking these Bangladeshi vegetarian and vegan delights!

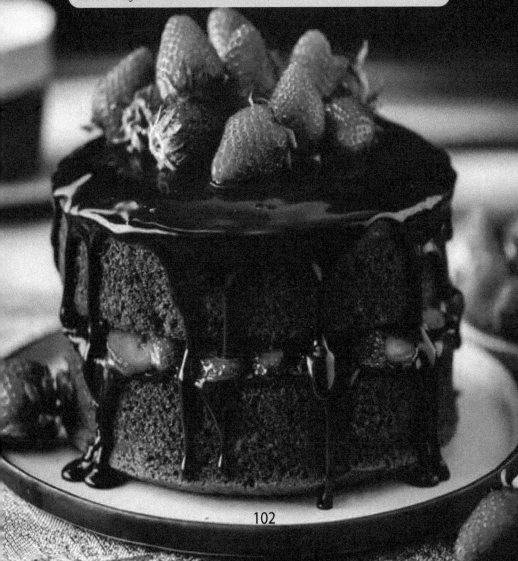

Chapter 8:

The Sweet Endings

No meal in Bangladesh is complete without a taste of something sweet. From rich, creamy sweets to refreshing, fruity desserts, Bangladeshi cuisine offers a delightful range of desserts to satisfy any sweet tooth. This chapter will guide you through the irresistible world of Bangladeshi desserts.

Mishti
The Milky Delights

Mishti, or sweetmeats, are a significant part of Bangladeshi culinary tradition. They are often made from milk, sugar, and ghee. 'Roshogolla', 'Mishti Doi' (sweet yogurt), and 'Chom Chom' are some beloved classics that are often served at festivities and celebrations.

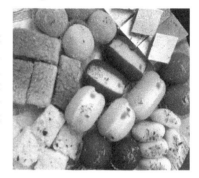

1. Roshogolla Recipe

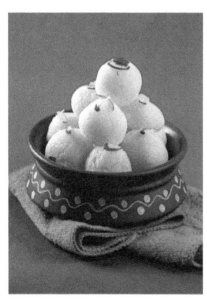

Ingredients:

- 1 liter whole milk
- 3 tablespoons lemon juice
- 1 cup sugar
- 4 cups water

Instructions:

1. Bring the milk to a boil in a heavy-bottomed pan. Once boiling, add the lemon juice to curdle the milk.

2. Strain the curdled milk through a muslin cloth. Rinse with cold water to remove the lemon's sourness and squeeze out the excess water.

3. Knead the milk solids (chhena) until smooth. Divide into small round balls.

4. In a large pan, bring the sugar and water to a boil to make the syrup.

5. Add the milk balls to the boiling syrup and cook for about 15 minutes until they double in size.

6. Let it cool down and then chill before serving. Certainly! Both Chom Chom (also known as Cham Cham) and Mishti Doi are delightful and popular Bengali sweets. Let's dive into the recipes:

2. Chom Chom (Cham Cham) Recipe

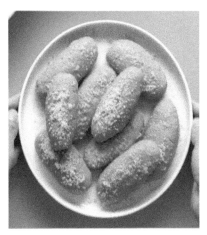

Ingredients:

For the Chom Chom:
1. 1 liter full-fat milk
2. 3 tbsp lemon juice (or vinegar)
3. 1 cup sugar
4. 4 cups water

For Garnishing:

1. 200g mawa or khoya (dried evaporated milk solids)
2. Some chopped pistachios or almonds
3. Saffron strands (optional)
4. A pinch of cardamom powder

Instructions:

1. Making Chhena (Paneer):

- Bring the milk to boil in a large pot. Once boiling, add the lemon juice or vinegar and stir until the milk curdles.
- Remove from heat and strain the curdled milk using a muslin cloth. Wash the chhena under cold water to remove the sourness of the lemon or vinegar. Tie and hang it for an hour to remove excess water.

2. Preparing the Chom Chom:

- Knead the chhena until smooth and soft. Divide and shape them into oval or cylindrical shapes.
- In a large pan, boil the sugar and water to make a syrup. Once boiling, gently drop the chhena rolls into the syrup. Cook for about 15-20 minutes on medium heat.
- Remove from heat and let them cool.

3. Garnishing:

- Roll the chom chom over grated mawa or khoya.
- Garnish with chopped pistachios, almonds, a pinch of cardamom powder, and saffron strands.

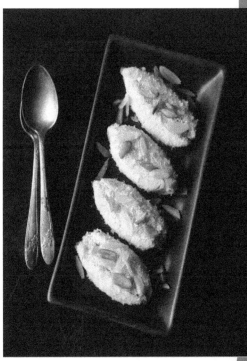

3. Mishti Doi (Sweet Yogurt) Recipe

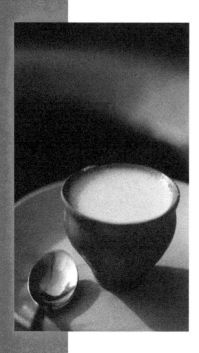

Ingredients:

1. 1 liter full-fat milk
2. 1/2 cup plain yogurt (curd) as a starter
3. 3/4 cup sugar (you can adjust to taste)

Instructions:

1. Caramelizing Sugar:

- In a pan, heat a portion (about 1/4 cup) of the sugar on low heat until it melts and turns a golden -brown caramel color. Be careful not to burn it.

2. Preparing Milk:

- In another pot, bring the milk to a boil. Simmer until it reduces to three-fourths of its original volume.
- Add the caramelized sugar to this milk and stir well. Allow it to cool to l

3. Setting the Yogurt:

- Once the milk is lukewarm, mix in the plain yogurt. Make sure to whisk it well to ensure even mixing.
- Transfer this mixture to a clay or earthen pot (traditionally used for Mishti Doi because it absorbs excess moisture, making the yogurt thick).
- Cover and place it in a warm, draft-free place for 8-12 hours or overnight. The yogurt should set and have a creamy consistency.
- Once set, refrigerate for a few hours before serving.

Serve the Mishti Doi chilled in the clay pot for an authentic experience!

Section 8.2:

Pitha – The Versatile Treats

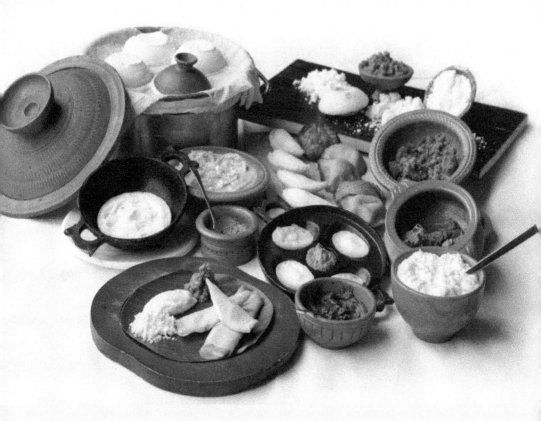

Pitha refers to a wide range of rice cakes and dumplings, which are often sweet but can also be savory. 'Bhapa Pitha' (steamed rice cake filled with jaggery), 'Puli Pitha' (dumplings filled with coconut), and 'Patishapta' (crepe-like pitha filled with milk solids) are a few examples of sweet pitha.

Bhapa Pitha Recipe

Ingredients:

- 2 cups rice flour
- 1 cup grated coconut
- 1 cup jaggery
- Salt to taste

Instructions:

1. Prepare a dough by adding a little water to the rice flour and a pinch of salt.
2. In a separate bowl, mix the grated coconut and jaggery.
3. Take a small portion of the dough and flatten it on your palm. Place a spoonful of the coconut-jaggery mixture in the center and fold the dough over it to form a half-moon shape. Seal the edges tightly.
4. Steam these pithas in a steamer for about 10-15 minutes until cooked.
5. Serve the Bhapa Pitha hot or cold as per preference.

Puli Pitha

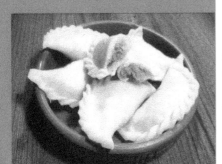

Puli Pitha, also known as "Dudh Puli" or simply "Puli," is a traditional Bengali sweet dish often prepared during the winter months and special occasions. It consists of rice dumplings with a filling of coconut and jaggery, cooked in a creamy milk sauce. Here's a recipe for Puli Pitha:

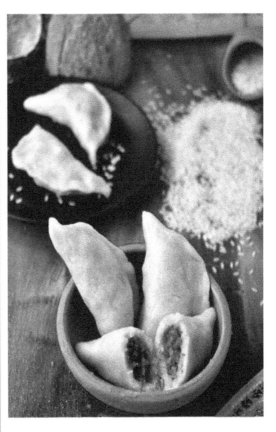

Ingredients:

For the Dough:
1. 1 cup rice flour
2. A pinch of salt
3. Hot water, as required

For the Filling:

1. 1 cup grated coconut
2. 1/2 cup jaggery or palm sugar (you can adjust the sweetness as per your preference)
3. 2-3 cardamom pods, seeds removed and crushed

For the Milk Sauce:

1. 2-3 cups of milk
2. 1/4 cup jaggery or sugar (or adjust to taste)
3. 1/2 tsp cardamom powder

Instructions:

1. Prepare the Dough:
- In a mixing bowl, add the rice flour and a pinch of salt. Gradually add hot water and knead to form a smooth dough. Cover it with a damp cloth and set it aside.

2. Prepare the Filling:
- In a pan, melt the jaggery over low heat. Once it's melted, add the grated coconut and cardamom. Mix well and cook until the mixture thickens. Remove from heat and let it cool.

3. Shape the Pithas:
- Take a small portion of the dough and make it into a ball. Flatten it with your fingers to form a small disc.
- Place a spoonful of the coconut-jaggery mixture in the center of the disc. Fold the dough to cover the filling and seal the edges to form a crescent shape or a half-moon. You can also make round or oval shapes.
- Repeat this process with the remaining dough and filling.

4. Prepare the Milk Sauce:
- In a large saucepan, bring the milk to a boil. Keep stirring occasionally to prevent it from sticking to the bottom. Reduce the heat and let it simmer until the milk is reduced to half its volume.
- Add jaggery or sugar and cardamom powder to the milk and stir well until the sweetener is dissolved.

5. Cook the Pithas:
- Gently drop the prepared pithas into the simmering milk. Let them cook for 10-15 minutes or until they are soft and fully cooked.
- Once done, remove from heat.

6. Serve:
- Serve Puli Pitha warm or let it cool down and serve it at room temperature. You can also refrigerate it and serve it chilled.

Note: The consistency of the milk sauce is up to your preference. Some like it thick and creamy, while others prefer a thinner consistency. Adjust the cooking time of the milk accordingly.

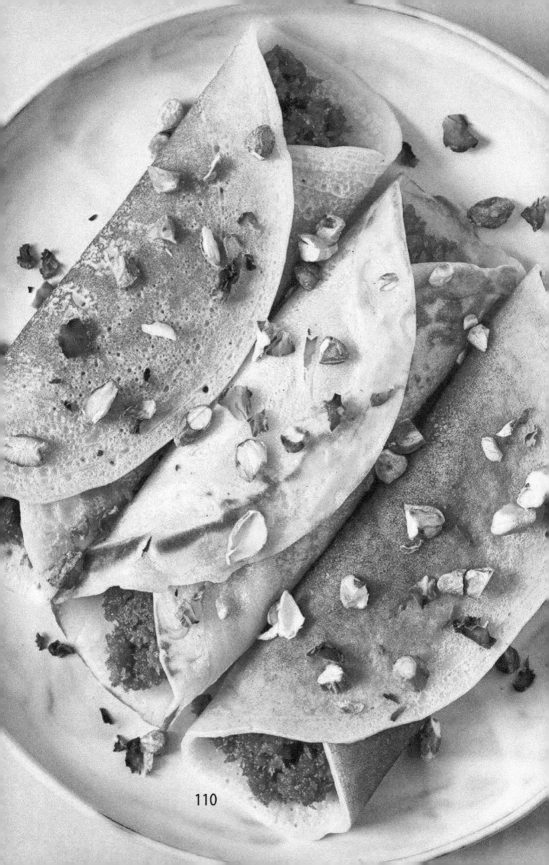

Patishapta

Patishapta is a popular Bengali dessert, particularly made during the winter months. It's essentially a thin rice flour crepe filled with a coconut and jaggery or khoya (reduced milk) mixture. Here's a traditional recipe for Patishapta:

Ingredients:

For the Crepes:

1. 1/2 cup rice flour
2. 1/4 cup refined flour (all-purpose flour)
3. 2 tbsp semolina (sooji)
4. 1 cup milk (or as required to make a thin batter)
5. A pinch of salt

For the Filling:

1. 1 cup grated coconut
2. 1/2 cup jaggery or palm sugar (adjust based on sweetness desired)
3. 1/2 cup khoya (reduced milk solids) - optional
4. 2-3 cardamom pods, seeds removed and crushed

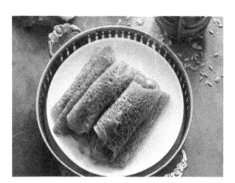

Instructions:

1. Prepare the Filling:

- In a pan, melt the jaggery over low heat.
- Once melted, add the grated coconut, khoya (if using), and crushed cardamom. Mix well.
- Cook the mixture until it becomes thick and leaves the sides of the pan. Remove from heat and set aside to cool.

2. Prepare the Crepe Batter:

- In a mixing bowl, combine the rice flour, refined flour, semolina, and a pinch of salt.
- Gradually add milk, mixing continuously, to form a smooth and runny batter. Ensure there are no lumps. The batter should be of pouring consistency, similar to that of pancake batter.

3. Make the Patishapta:

- Heat a non-stick skillet or tawa over medium heat. Brush it with a little ghee or oil.
- Pour a ladleful of the batter on the skillet and spread it into a thin circle, similar to making a pancake or crepe.
- Once tiny bubbles appear on the surface, place a portion of the filling on one side of the crepe.
- Gently roll the crepe to cover the filling, similar to making a wrap or roll. Let it cook for another minute until it's golden and crispy on the edges.
- Remove from the skillet and place on a serving plate.

4. Serve:

- Patishapta is traditionally served warm, often drizzled with condensed milk or a thickened milk sauce.

HALWA - THE COMFORTING DESSERTS

Halwa, in various forms, is a beloved dessert across the vast swathes of the subcontinent. These thick, often gelatinous, sweet dishes are made by simmering ingredients in milk or water and sweetening them with sugar. The addition of ghee, cardamom, and various nuts make them a fragrant and indulgent treat. In Bangladesh, a couple of halwas stand out due to their unique texture and taste. Let's delve into one of the most cherished ones: Suji (Semolina) Halwa.

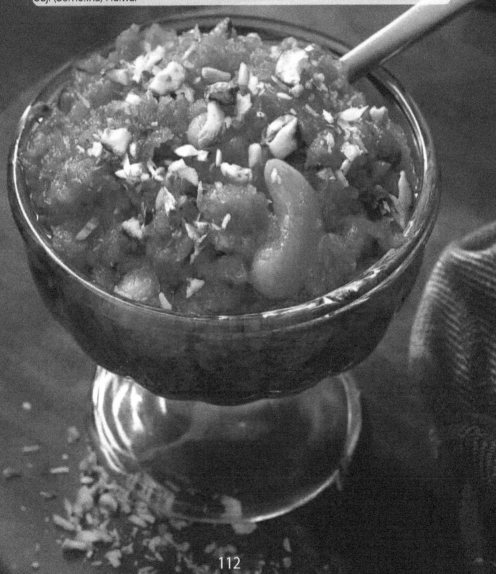

Suji Halwa

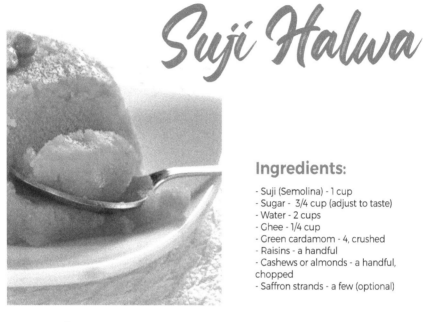

Ingredients:

- Suji (Semolina) - 1 cup
- Sugar - 3/4 cup (adjust to taste)
- Water - 2 cups
- Ghee - 1/4 cup
- Green cardamom - 4, crushed
- Raisins - a handful
- Cashews or almonds - a handful, chopped
- Saffron strands - a few (optional)

Instructions:

1. In a heavy-bottomed pan, heat the ghee on medium flame.
2. Add the semolina and roast it, stirring continuously to ensure it doesn't burn. Roast until it turns a light golden color and emits a nutty aroma.
3. In a separate pan, boil the water with sugar, crushedcardamom, and saffron strands. Stir until the sugar dissolves completely. Turn off the heat once it comes to a boil.
4. Slowly add this sugar-water mixture to the roasted semolina, stirring continuously to avoid forming lumps.
5. Keep stirring until the mixture thickens and starts leaving the sides of the pan.
6. Toss in the raisins and the chopped nuts. **Mix well**.
7. Transfer the halwa to a serving dish and garnish with a few more nuts or saffron strands.
8. Serve warm.

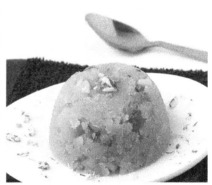

Culinary Note: Suji Halwa can be served on its own or accompanied by puris (deep-fried Indian bread) during special occasions. The gentle cardamom scent combined with the rich taste of ghee and the crunch of nuts makes this a comforting dessert, perfect for cold evenings or festive celebrations.Other popular variations of halwa in Bangladeshi cuisine include Carrot Halwa and Lentil Halwa. Each variant offers a unique taste and texture, but all are united by their rich, comforting sweetness.

113

Section 8.4:
Seasonal Fruits–
The Natural Sweets

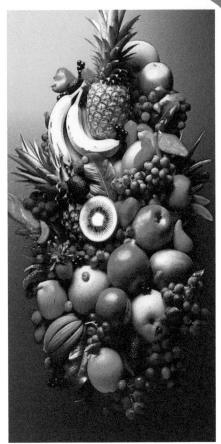

Bangladesh, with its tropical climate, offers a wealth of fresh fruits that often serve as a light and refreshing end to meals. Mango, jackfruit, and lychee are popular fruits, often served fresh or in simple desserts like 'Aam Doi' (mango yogurt) .

Aam Doi Recipe

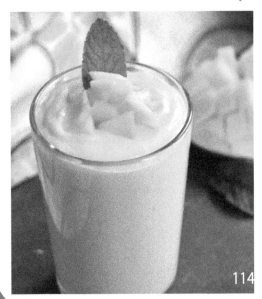

Ingredients:

- 2 ripe mangoes
- 2 cups yogurt
- 1 cup condensed milk
- 1/2 cup sugar

Instructions:

1. Peel and puree the mangoes.
2. Mix the yogurt, condensed milk, and sugar until smooth. Add the mango puree and mix well.
3. Pour the mixture into an oven-safe bowl.
4. Preheat the oven to 180°C (350°F) and bake the yogurt mixture for about 15-20 minutes, or until it sets.
5. Allow it to cool and then refrigerate before serving the Aam Doi.

Section 8.5:
Traditional
Bangladeshi *Drinks*

Bangladesh has a variety of traditional sweet beverages that are often enjoyed at the end of a meal. **'Borhani'**, a savory-sweet yogurt drink, and 'Lassi', a sweet and creamy yogurt-based drink, are favorites during the hot months, while **'Cha'** (tea) flavored with cardamom or ginger is a comforting choice for colder weather.

Sweet endings in Bangladeshi cuisine range from the traditionally rich and decadent to the refreshingly simple and fruity, ensuring there's a dessert for every palate. These desserts not only provide a satisfying end to a meal but also offer a sweet glimpse into the country's rich cultural and culinary heritage. As we journey on, we will explore the influence of international flavors on Bangladeshi cuisine and how it has adapted and embraced these influences.

Chapter 9: The Art of Bangladeshi Beverage

From the ubiquitous tea to refreshing sherbets, beverages play a pivotal role in Bangladeshi cuisine. They not only serve to cleanse the palate and aid digestion but also provide an opportunity to experience an array of flavors that accompany and complete a traditional Bangladeshi meal. This chapter will guide you through the fascinating world of **Bangladeshi beverages**.

Section 9.1:
Cha - The National Drink

Tea, or 'Cha', is the national drink of Bangladesh. It is consumed throughout the day and during any occasion. 'Bengal Milk Tea', a rich and creamy concoction, and 'Masala Cha', infused with a blend of aromatic spices, are two variations of this national favorite.

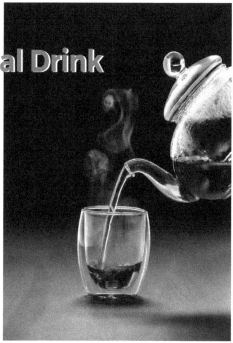

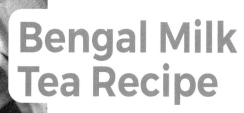

Bengal Milk Tea Recipe

Ingredients:

- 2 cups water
- 2 teaspoons loose black tea
- 1-2 tablespoons sugar
- 1 cup milk

Instructions:

1. Boil the water in a pot. Add the loose black tea and sugar, then simmer for a few minutes.
2. Add the milk and bring to a boil, then reduce heat and let it simmer for 2-3 minutes.
3. Strain the tea into cups and serve hot.

It seems you're asking about **Masala Chai,** a popular spiced tea that's enjoyed in various parts of India and has gained **international** recognition. Here's a classic recipe for **Masala Chai:**

Masala Chai
(Spiced Tea) Recipe

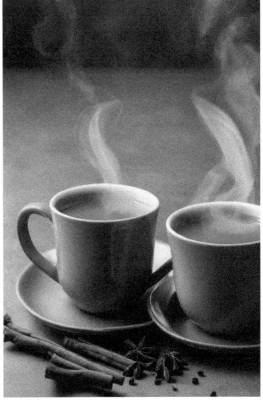

Ingredients:

1. Tea:

- 2 cups of water
- 1 to 2 tablespoons of black tea leaves (or 2-3 tea bags)
- 1 to 1.5 cups of milk (preferably whole milk for a richer flavor)

2. Spices (adjust according to prefer ence):

- 2-4 green cardamom pods (crushed)
- 1-inch piece of cinnamon stick
- 2-4 cloves
- 1/2-inch piece of ginger (crushed or grated)
- A pinch of black pepper (optional)
- 1/2 tsp of fennel seeds (optional)

3. Sweetener:

- Sugar or jaggery to taste (typically 2-3 teaspoons, but adjust according to your preference)

Instructions:

1. Prepare Spices: Crush the cardamom, cloves, and ginger. If you like your chai more aromatic and spicier, you can also crush the cinnamon and fennel seeds.

2. Boil Water: In a pot, bring the 2 cups of water to a boil.

3. Add Spices: Add the crushed spices to the boiling water. Allow the spices to steep and infuse for about 2-3 minutes on medium heat. This releases their flavor into the water.

4. Add Tea: Introduce the tea leaves or tea bags to the pot. Let it brew for 1-2 minutes. The longer you brew, the stronger the tea will be.

5. Pour in Milk: Add the milk to the pot. Depending on how milky you like your chai, you can adjust the quantity. Bring the mixture back to a boil.

6. Sweeten: Add sugar or jaggery according to taste. Allow the tea to simmer for another 2 -3 minutes, stirring occasionally.

7. Strain & Serve: Strain the tea to remove the tea leaves and spices. Pour the masala chai into cups and serve hot.

Tips:

- The amount and variety of spices can be adjusted based on personal preferences. Some people may prefer a stronger ginger flavor, while others might like the sweet aroma of cardamom.
- Masala chai can also be brewed using a combination of different teas, such as Assam, Darjeeling, or Ceylon.

Enjoy your warm, aromatic, and comforting cup of Masala Chai!

The Refreshing Yogurt Drinks

' Lassi' and 'Doi Sharbat' are both yogurt-based beverages enjoyed particularly during the hot summer months. They are creamy, refreshing and can be either sweet, often flavored with ripe mangoes or strawberries, or savory, spiced with a hint of cumin and salt.

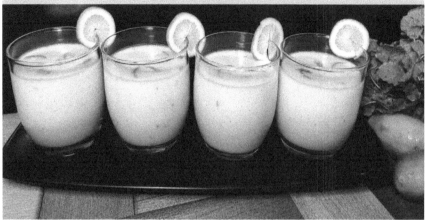

Mango Lassi Recipe

Ingredients:

- 2 ripe mangoes
- 2 cups plain yogurt
- 2 tablespoons sugar
- 1 cup cold water or milk
- Ice cubes

Instructions:

1. Peel and chop the mangoes.
2. Blend the chopped mangoes, yogurt, sugar, and water (or milk) until smooth.
3. Pour the lassi into glasses, add some ice cubes, and serve chilled.

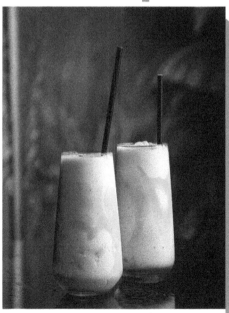

Borhani - The Traditional Digestive

'Borhani' is a savory drink made from yogurt and a unique blend of spices like mint, coriander, and mustard. It is traditionally served at weddings and special occasions and is believed to aid digestion

Borhani Recipe

Ingredients:

- 2 cups yogurt
- 1 teaspoon black salt
- 1 teaspoon roasted cumin powder
- 1 teaspoon mint leaves paste
- 1 teaspoon coriander leaves paste
- 1/2 teaspoon black pepper
- 1/2 teaspoon mustard
- Salt to taste

Instructions:

1. Blend all the ingredients together until smooth.
2. Chill the Borhani in the refrigerator for a few hours before serving.

Section 9.4:

Fruit Juices and
Sherbets

Bangladesh's tropical climate offers a variety of fruits that are often turned into refreshing juices and sherbets. 'Aam Panna' (a tangy drink made from green mangoes), 'Bel Sherbet' (wood apple sherbet), and 'Lemur Sharbat' (lime sherbet) are just a few of the many refreshing fruit-based beverages.

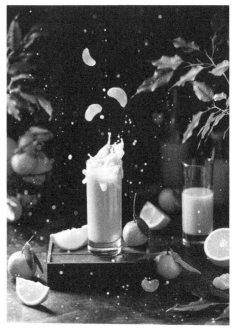

Aam Panna Recipe

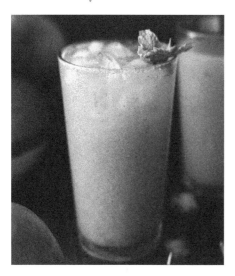

Ingredients:

- 2 raw mangoes
- 4 cups water
- 1 cup sugar
- 1 teaspoon black salt
- 1 teaspoon roasted cumin powder
- Mint leaves for garnish

Instructions:

1. Boil the raw mangoes in water until they become soft and pulpy. Let them cool.
2. Peel the mangoes and extract the pulp.
3. Blend the pulp with water, sugar, black salt, and roasted cumin powder until smooth.
4. Pour the Aam Panna into glasses, garnish with mint leaves, and serve chilled.

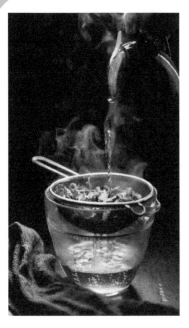

Section 9.5: Herbal Drinks and Infusions

The therapeutic properties of herbs have been cherished by the people of Bangladesh for ages. These humble plants not only elevate the flavor of our dishes but also infuse our beverages with medicinal benefits. Let's explore a couple of the traditional herbal infusions enjoyed in Bangladesh.

Tulsi Tea

Ingredients:

- Tulsi (holy basil) leaves - 10-12
- Water - 2 cups
- Honey - 1 tsp (adjust to taste)
- Lemon slice - 1
- Ginger (optional) - a small slice

Instructions:

1. Begin by boiling the water in a pot.
2. Add the tulsi leaves and ginger slice to the boiling water.
3. Let it simmer for 5-7 minutes, allowing the essence of tulsi and ginger to seep into the water.
4. Turn off the heat and strain the tea into a cup.
5. Add honey according to taste and stir well. Garnish with a slice of lemon.
6. Serve hot and enjoy the soothing properties of the tea.

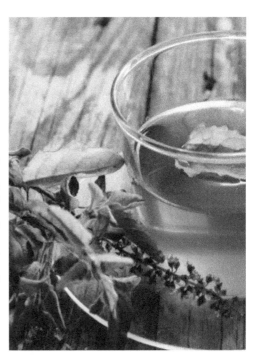

Lemongrass-Ginger Sherbet

Ingredients:

- Lemongrass stalks - 2, roughly chopped
- Ginger - 1-inch piece, sliced
- Water - 4 cups
- Sugar - 1/2 cup (adjust to taste)
- Lemon juice - 2 tbsp

Instructions:

1. Combine the lemongrass, ginger, and water in a pot.

2. Bring the mixture to a boil, then reduce the heat and let it simmer for about 10 minutes.

3. Add sugar and stir until it completely dissolves.

4. Turn off the heat and allow the mixture to cool down.

5. Once cooled, strain out the lemongrass and ginger pieces.

6. Add lemon juice to the infusion and mix well.

7. Serve chilled, preferably with ice cubes.

Culinary Note: These drinks are not only refreshing but also pack a range of health benefits. Tulsi, for instance, is known to boost immunity, improve digestion, and combat respiratory ailments. Ginger, on the other hand, is a potent remedy for coughs, colds, and digestion issues. Embracing the tradition of herbal infusions is like journeying through the annals of Bangladeshi heritage. These beverages encapsulate the essence of the land, the wisdom of ancestors, and the love for nature in every sip.

Chapter 10:

The *Celebration* Foods

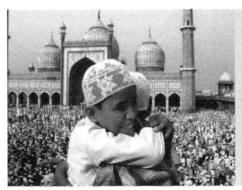

In Bangladeshi culture, food is central to celebrations. Be it a religious festival, a wedding, or a family gathering, the occasion is marked with an array of traditional dishes that are rich in flavor and steeped in history. This chapter explores these special dishes, allowing you to create your own festive Bangladeshi feast, wherever you may be.

Section 10.1: Eid Delicacies

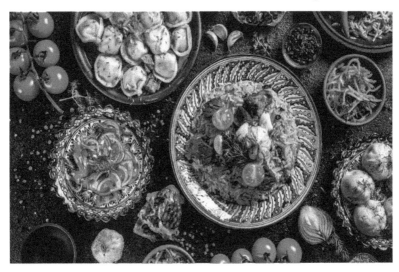

Eid, a major Muslim festival, is celebrated with a variety of special dishes. 'Biryani' and 'Korma' often take center stage, accompanied by 'Sheer Khurma' (a vermicelli pudding with dates and nuts) and 'Firni' (rice flour pudding).

Chicken Biryani
(Eid Delicacy)

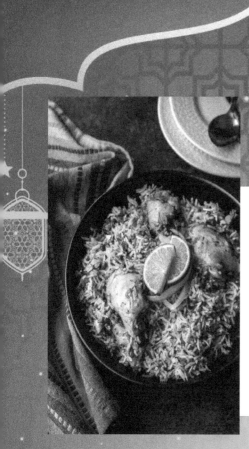

Ingredients:
- 2 cups Basmati rice
- 500g chicken, cut into pieces
- 2 onions, finely sliced
- 2 tomatoes, chopped
- 2 tablespoons ginger-garlic paste
- 2 green chilies, slit
- 1 cup plain yogurt
- 1 teaspoon turmeric powder
- 1 teaspoon red chili powder
- 2 teaspoons Biryani masala
- 4 cups water
- Salt to taste
- 3 tablespoons oil
- Handful of fresh mint and coriander
  leaves

Steps:

1. Rinse the basmati rice under cold water until the water runs clear. Soak the rice in water for 30 minutes, then drain and set aside.

2. Heat oil in a large pot over medium heat. Add the sliced onions and sauté until golden brown.

3. Add the ginger-garlic paste and green chilies. Sauté for a few more minutes until the raw smell disappears.

4. Add the chopped tomatoes, turmeric powder, red chili powder, and Biryani masala. Cook until the tomatoes are soft and the spices are well blended.

5. Add the chicken pieces to the pot and cook until they are well coated with the spices and partially cooked.

6. Stir in the yogurt, cover the pot, and cook on low heat for about 10 minutes.

7. In a separate pot, bring 4 cups of water to a boil. Add the soaked and drained basmati rice to the boiling water. Cook the rice until it's 70% cooked, then drain the water.

8. Layer the partially cooked rice over the chicken in the pot. Sprinkle the fresh mint and coriander leaves on top. Cover the pot with a tight lid.

9. Cook on low heat for about 30 minutes, until the rice is fully cooked and has absorbed the flavors of the chicken and spices.

10. Serve the Biryani hot, with a side of raita or hard-boiled eggs.

Sheer Khurma Recipe

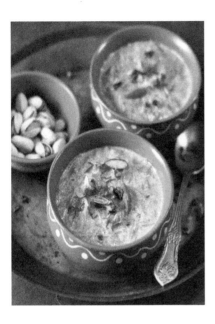

Ingredients:

1. cup of vermicelli — 1
2. cups of full-fat milk — 4
3. cup of sugar — 1/2
4. dates (chopped) — 10-12
5. cup of mixed nuts
   (almonds, pistachios, cashews) — 1/2
6. teaspoon of cardamom powder — 1/2
7. tablespoons of ghee — 2

Instructions:

1. Heat the ghee in a large pan, add the vermicelli and fry until golden brown.
2. Add the milk and bring it to boil. Simmer the heat and let it cook until the vermicelli is soft.
3. Add the sugar, dates, nuts, and cardamom powder, and cook for another 10-15 minutes until everything is well combined.
4. Serve hot or chilled, garnished with some more nuts.

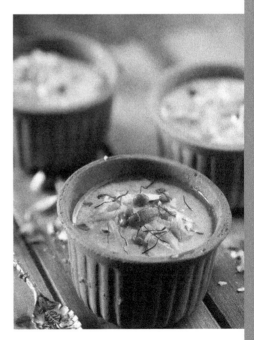

Firni (or Phirni) is a classic North Indian dessert made with ground rice, milk, sugar, and flavored with cardamom, saffron, and rose water. It's traditionally served in clay pots and is a popular treat during festivals and special occasions. Here's a recipe for Firni:

Firni (Rice Flour Pudding) Recipe

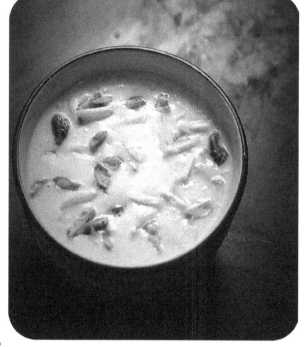

Ingredients:

1. 1/4 cup basmati rice **(or rice ofchoice)**
2. 1 liter full-fat milk
3. 1/2 to 3/4 cup sugar **(adjust to taste)**
4. 1/2 tsp cardamom powder
5. A pinch of saffron strands **(optional)**
6. 1 tbsp rose water **(optional)**
7. Chopped nuts like almonds, pistachios, or cashews for garnishing
8. Silver leaf **(varak)** for decoration **(optional)**

Instructions:

1. Prepare Rice:
- Wash the rice thoroughly and soak it in water for about 30 minutes.
- Drain the water and grind the rice into a coarse paste. A little water can be added to facilitate grinding, but the paste should be thick.

2. Cooking the Firni:
- In a heavy-bottomed pan or pot, bring the milk to a boil. Reduce the heat to medium.
- Gradually add the ground rice paste to the milk, stirring continuously to prevent lumps from forming.
- Keep stirring and cook on low to medium heat until the rice is fully cooked and the mixture thickens.

3. Adding Sweetness and Flavor:
- Add sugar to the thickened milk and rice mixture. Stir well until the sugar is fully dissolved.
- Introduce the cardamom powder, saffron strands, and rose water (if using). Mix well.

4. Final Steps and Serving:
- Once the firni reaches your desired consistency (remember, it thickens more as it cools), remove it from heat.
- Pour the firni into individual clay pots or serving bowls. Allow it to cool to room temperature.
- Refrigerate for a few hours until set.
- Before serving, garnish with chopped nuts and, if desired, a piece of silver leaf.

Notes:
- The consistency of Firni is creamy and a bit grainy, which differentiates it from other rice puddings.
- You can also add fruit purees (like mango) to make different flavored Firni.
Serve your Firni chilled and enjoy this creamy, luscious dessert with family and friends!

Pohela Boishakh – Bangladeshi New Year Foods

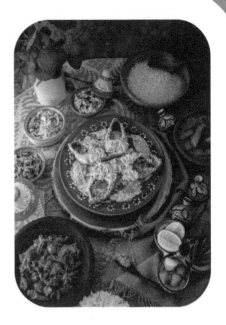

Pohela Boishakh, the Bengali New Year, is welcomed with traditional foods such as 'Panta Bhat' (fermented rice), 'Hilsa Fish', and an assortment of 'Pithas'. 'Payesh' (rice pudding) is also commonly prepared as a dessert.

Panta Bhat Recipe

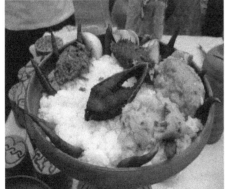

Ingredients:

1. 1 cup of rice
2. Water
3. Salt (to taste)

Instructions:

1. Cook the rice as you usually would, but make it a bit softer than usual.
2. Once cooked, let the rice cool down, then add enough water to fully submerge the rice.
3. Cover and let it sit at room temperature for about 24 hours to ferment.
4. After 24 hours, the Panta Bhat is ready. It is typically served cold with salt, green chilies, and a wedge of lemon.

Section 10.3:
Wedding Feasts

Bangladeshi weddings are known for their lavish feasts. 'Mutton Kacchi Biryani', 'Chicken Roast', 'Shorshe Ilish' (Hilsa in mustard sauce), and 'Mishti' (sweets) are some of the dishes usually served.

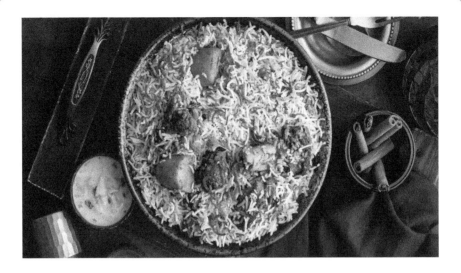

Mutton Kacchi Biryani Recipe

Ingredients:

1. 500g mutton, cut into pieces
2. 2 cups basmati rice
3. 2 onions, finely sliced
4. 2 tablespoons ginger-garlic paste
5. 1 cup yogurt
6. 1 teaspoon turmeric powder
7. 1 teaspoon red chili powder
8. 1 teaspoon Biryani masala
9. Salt to taste
10. 4 cups water
11. 3 tablespoons oil or ghee

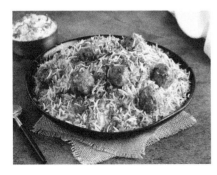

Instructions:

1. Marinate the mutton with ginger-garlic paste, yogurt, turmeric powder, red chili powder, Biryani masala, and salt. Let it sit for at least 2 hours.

2. In a large pan, heat the oil or ghee and sauté the onions until golden brown.

3. Add the marinated mutton and cook on a low flame until the mutton is tender.

4. In a separate pot, boil the water, add a bit of salt and cook the rice until it's 70% done.

5. Drain the water and layer the partially cooked rice over the mutton in the pan.

6. Cover the pan with a tight lid and cook on a very low flame for about 30-40 minutes until the rice is fully cooked and has absorbed the flavors from the mutton.

7. Mix gently and serve hot with raita and salad.

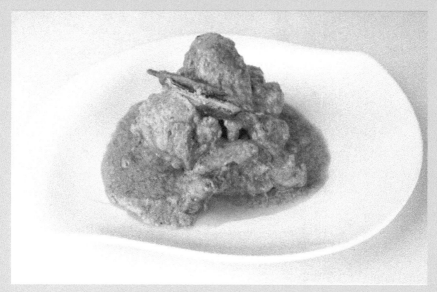

Chicken Roast

The Bangladeshi Chicken Roast, often referred to as "Chicken Roast" in local parlance, is not your typical oven roast. It is a rich, spiced chicken dish, slow-cooked in a thick gravy, often served during special occasions and festive times. Here's how you can make this delectable dish at home:

Ingredients:

- **Chicken:** ....1 whole (approx. 1.5 kg), cleaned and cut intopieces
- **Yogurt:** ....1 cup
- **Onion:** ....2 large, finely sliced
- **Ginger paste:** ....2 tsp
- **Garlic paste:** ....2 tsp
- **Red chili powder:** ....1 tsp
- **Turmeric powder:** ....1/2 tsp
- **Cumin powder:** ....1/2 tsp

- **Coriander powder:** ....1/2 tsp
- **Green chilies:** ....4-6, slit
- **Bay leaves:** 2
- **Cinnamon sticks:** 2
- **Cardamom pods:** 4-5
- **Cloves:** 4-5
- **Star anise:** 1
- **Ghee or cooking oil:** ....1/2 cup
- **Salt:** ....to taste
- **Sugar:** ....1 tsp
- **Lemon juice:** ....2 tbsp
- **Fresh coriander leaves:** ....for garnishing

Instructions:

1. *Marination:* In a large bowl, mix yogurt, ginger paste, garlic paste, red chili powder, turmeric powder, cumin powder, coriander powder, salt, and half of the lemon juice. Add the chicken pieces, ensuring they are well-coated with the marinade. Let it sit for at least 2 hours, preferably overnight in the refrigerator.

2. In a large pot or pan, heat ghee or oil. Add the sugar and let it caramelize to give the roast its signature reddish-brown color.

3. Add the bay leaves, cinnamon sticks, cardamom pods, cloves, and star anise. Sauté for a minute until aromatic.

4. Add the finely sliced onions and fry until they become golden brown.

5. Reduce the heat and add the marinated chicken pieces. Mix well to ensure the chicken is covered with the onions and spices.

6. Cover and cook on low heat. The chicken will release its juices.

7. When the chicken is half-cooked, add the slit green chilies.

8. Continue cooking on low heat until the chicken is fully cooked and tender. The gravy should be thick and rich, and the oil/ghee will start to separate from the sides.

9. Finish with the remaining lemon juice for a hint of tang.

10. Garnish with fresh coriander leaves.

11. Serve hot with pulao, naan, or paratha.

Culinary Note: Bangladeshi Chicken Roast is known for its rich and spicy flavor. The dish beautifully balances heat, tanginess, and sweetness. Adjust the level of spiciness as per your preference. The key to a perfect chicken roast is slow cooking, allowing the chicken to absorb all the flavors.

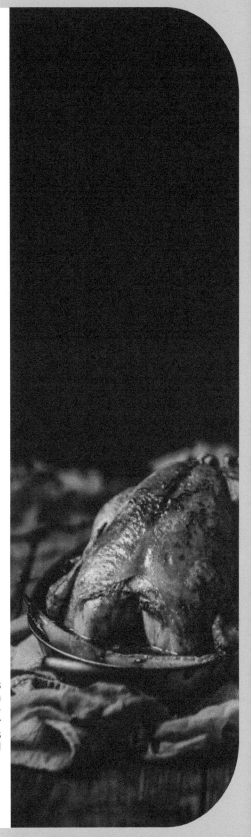

Puja Prasad

Hindu Festive Foods

During Hindu festivals like Durga Puja and Saraswati Puja, vegetarian dishes are prepared as **'Prasad'** (a religious offering). **'Khichuri'** (a dish made from rice and lentils), **'Labra'** (mixed vegetable curry), and sweet treats like 'Rosogolla' and 'Sandesh' are common.

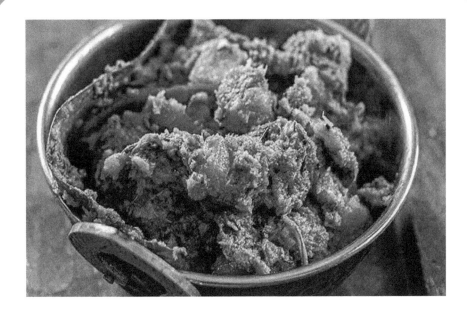

1. Labra
(Bengali Mixed Vegetable Curry)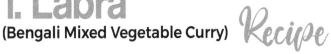

Ingredients:

1. Mixed vegetables of choice: 1 cup pumpkin (cubed), 1 cup eggplant (cubed), 1 potato (cubed), 1/2 cup radish (sliced), 1/2 cup green beans (chopped), 1/2 cup cauliflower florets, etc.

2. 1/2 tsp fenugreek seeds (methi seeds)

3. 1 tsp cumin seeds

4. 2-3 dried red chilies

5. 1 bay leaf

6. 1 tsp turmeric powder

7. 1 tsp cumin powder

8. 1 tsp red chili powder (adjust to taste)

9. Salt to taste

10. 1 tsp sugar

11. 2 tbsp mustard oil (or any cooking oil)

12. A handful of fresh cilantro (coriander) leaves for garnishing

Instructions:

1. In a large pot or pan, heat mustard oil.

2. Add fenugreek seeds, cumin seeds, dried red chilies, and bay leaf. Sauté until they release their aroma.

3. Add all the mixed vegetables to the pot. Stir and sauté for 5-7 minutes.

4. Add turmeric powder, cumin powder, red chili powder, salt, and sugar. Mix well so that the spices coat all the vegetables.

5. Cover the pot and let it cook on low heat. The vegetables will release their moisture and cook in their juices.

6. Check occasionally and stir. If necessary, you can add a little water to prevent sticking.

7. Cook until all the vegetables are tender and the flavors meld together.

8. Adjust seasoning if necessary. Garnish with fresh cilantro.

9. Serve hot with rice or chapati.

Enjoy your warm, aromatic, and comforting cup of Masala Chai!

2. Sandesh
(Bengali Sweet)
Recipe

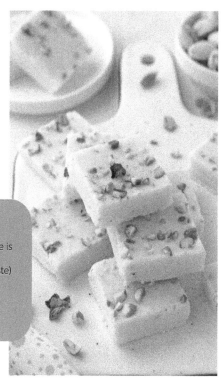

Ingredients:

1. 2 cups chhena (paneer) - freshly made is preferable
2. 1/2 cup powdered sugar (adjust to taste)
3. A pinch of cardamom powder
4. Saffron strands (optional)
5. Chopped pistachios or almonds for garnishing

Instructions:

1. Start by preparing chhena or paneer. (You can make this by boiling milk, adding lemon juice or vinegar to curdle it, and then draining and rinsing the curdled milk to obtain chhena.)

2. Place the chhena on a flat surface and knead it well for about 5-7 minutes until it becomes smooth.

3. In a non-stick pan, over low heat, add the kneaded chhena and powdered sugar. Cook while stirring continuously until the mixture leaves the sides of the pan.

4. Turn off the heat and mix in the cardamom powder. Allow the mixture to cool slightly.

5. Once the mixture is cool enough to handle but still warm, divide and shape it into small balls or discs. You can also use molds to shape the Sandesh.

6. Garnish each Sandesh with saffron strands and/or chopped nuts.

7. Allow them to cool completely and set. Refrigerate for a while before serving.

Serve Sandesh chilled as a delightful sweet treat after your meal!

Section 10.5:
Winter Delights

Winter in Bangladesh brings with it a bounty of fresh produce and a range of special dishes. **'Pithe'** (rice cakes) made from **'Nolen Gur'** (date palm jaggery), 'Makha Sandesh' (handmade milk fudge), and 'Paesh' (rice pudding) made with winter harvest rice are traditional favorites.

These special occasion and festival foods are a testament to the rich culinary heritage of Bangladesh. They bring people together in celebration, carrying forward traditions and creating memories. As we conclude this book in the next chapter, we will reflect on the journey and the exploration of Bangladeshi cuisine and its profound role in uniting people and preserving culture.

Pithe with
Nolen Gur
(Date Palm Jaggery Rice Cakes)

Ingredients:
- Rice flour: 2 cups
- Nolen Gur (date palm jaggery): 1 cup, grated
- Grated coconut: 1 cup
- Water: As needed
- Pinch of salt

Instructions:

1. For the filling, in a pan, melt half of the Nolen Gur over low heat until it becomes liquid.

2. Add the grated coconut and mix well. Cook until the mixture thickens and then set it aside.

3. In a separate bowl, mix the rice flour with water and a pinch of salt to make a smooth dough.

4. Take small portions of the dough, flatten them, and add the coconut-jaggery mixture in the center. Seal the edges to form a dumpling.

5. Steam these dumplings until they are cooked through.

6. Serve warm, drizzled with melted Nolen Gur.

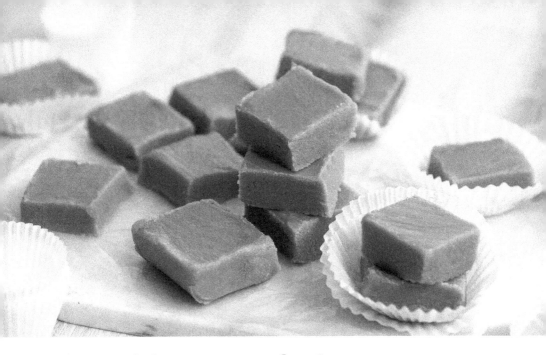

Makha Sandesh
(Handmade Milk Fudge)

Ingredients:

- Full-fat milk: 1 liter
- Lemon juice: 2 tbsp
- Sugar: 1/2 cup
- Cardamom powder: 1/4 tsp

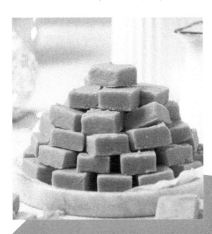

Instructions:

1. Boil milk in a heavy-bottomed pan. Once boiling, add lemon juice.
2. Stir gently until the milk curdles.
3. Drain the curdled milk to separate the whey and collect the milk solids (chhena).
4. Mash the chhena until smooth, and then cook it with sugar until the mixture thickens.
5. Add cardamom powder and mix well.
6. Remove from heat, and while still warm, shape into small patties.
7. Let them cool completely before serving.

Paesh

(Winter Harvest Rice Pudding)

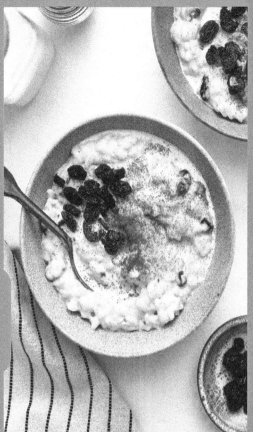

Ingredients:
- Winter harvest rice (preferably Gobindobhog rice): 1/2 cup
- Full-fat milk: 1 liter
- Sugar: 3/4 cup (adjust as per taste)
- Cardamom pods: 3-4
- Cashew nuts and raisins for garnishing

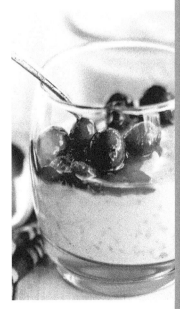

Instructions:

1. Wash the rice thoroughly and soak for 30 minutes.

2. In a large, heavy-bottomed pan, boil the milk.

3. Once boiling, reduce the heat and add the soaked rice.

4. Cook on low heat, stirring occasionally to prevent sticking.

5. When the rice is fully cooked and the milk has thickened, add sugar and cardamom pods.

6. Continue to cook for another 10 minutes.

7. Garnish with cashew nuts and raisins.

8. Serve warm or chilled, as preferred.

As winter wraps its cozy arms around Bangladesh, these dishes capture the essence of the season, and the love and warmth with which they're prepared and shared make them even more special. Their traditional roots run deep, and they embody the richness of Bangladeshi culture and culinary heritage. Whether it's the sweet allure of Pithe or the creamy comfort of Paesh, these dishes are a celebration of winter's bounty and the joy of festivity.

Chittagong Traditional Recipes

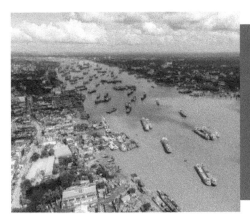

The port city of Chittagong, situated in southeastern Bangladesh, has its unique culinary flair influenced by the coastal geography and diverse ethnic communities. Here's a taste of Chittagong's distinct culinary offerings.

1. Mezban Beef Curry (Mezbani Ghosht)

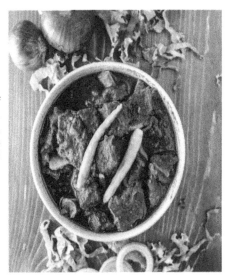

The Mezban, or Mezbani, is a traditional beef feast of the Chittagong region in Bangladesh. Mezbani beef curry is distinctively flavorful, spicy, and is an integral part of the region's cultural heritage. Here's a recipe for the famed Mezban Beef Curry:

Ingredients:

- **Beef:** 1 kg, cut into medium-sized pieces
- **Onion:** 2 large, finely sliced
- **Ginger paste:** 2 tablespoons
- **Garlic paste:** 2 tablespoons
- **Red chili powder:** 3-4 tablespoons (adjust to taste)
- **Turmeric powder:** 1 teaspoon
- **Coriander powder:** 1 tablespoon
- **Cumin powder:** 1 tablespoon
- **Garam masala powder:** 2 teaspoons
- **Mustard oil:** 1 cup
- **Salt:** to taste
- **Black pepper powder:** 1 teaspoon
- **Green chilies:** 6-8, slit
- **Roasted cumin powder:** 1 teaspoon
- **Roasted coriander powder:** 1 teaspoon
- **Tomato:** 2 large, finely chopped
- **Lemon juice:** 2 tablespoons
- **Coriander leaves:** a handful, chopped (for garnish)
- **Water:** as needed

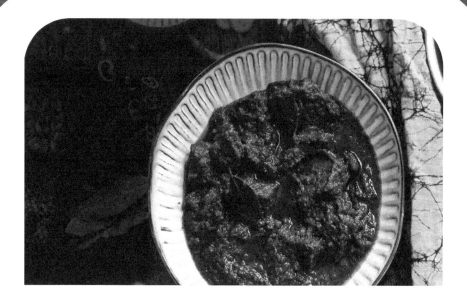

Directions:

1. Marination: Marinate the beef pieces with ginger paste, garlic paste, salt, lemon juice, and half of the red chili powder. Let it sit for at least 2 hours or overnight for better results.

2. In a heavy-bottomed pot or pan, heat the mustard oil until it reaches its smoking point. Reduce the flame to medium and add the sliced onions. Fry them until they're golden brown.

3. Add the marinated beef to the pan and fry on high heat until the beef is well-seared and browned on all sides.

4. Add chopped tomatoes and cook till they soften and become pulpy.

5. Add the rest of the red chili powder, turmeric powder, cumin powder, coriander powder, black pepper, and salt. Mix well and cook until oil starts separating from the masala.

6. Add water according to the consistency you desire for the curry. Generally, Mezbani Ghosht has a thick gravy. Bring the mixture to a boil, then reduce the flame to low and let it simmer.

7. Cover and cook on low heat until the beef is tender and the gravy is rich and flavorful.

8. Add garam masala, roasted cumin powder, roasted coriander powder, and slit green chilies. Mix well and let it simmer for another 10 minutes.

9. Once done, turn off the flame and let the curry sit for a while for the flavors to meld together.

10. Garnish with chopped coriander leaves before serving.

Serve the *Mezbani Ghosht* with plain rice or naan, and experience the rich flavors of *Chittagong*. Adjust the level of spices according to your preference. Remember, traditionally, this dish is quite *spicy!*

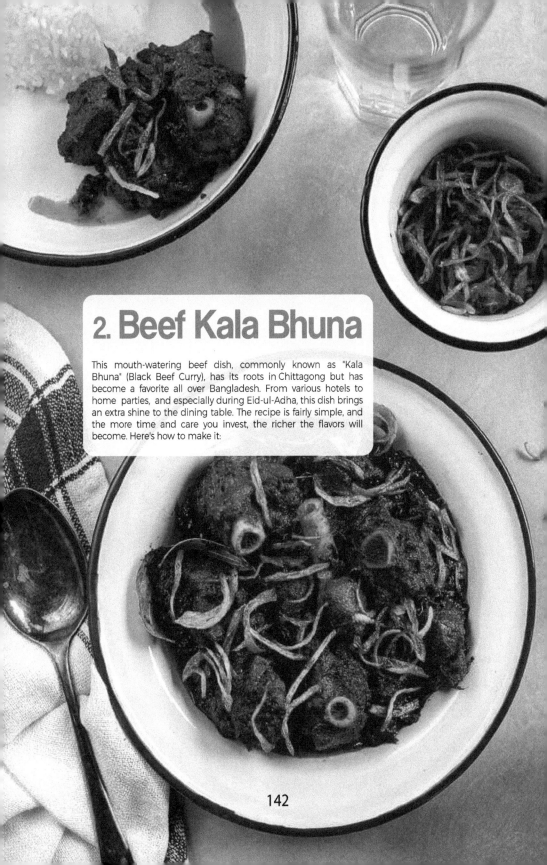

2. Beef Kala Bhuna

This mouth-watering beef dish, commonly known as "Kala Bhuna" (Black Beef Curry), has its roots in Chittagong but has become a favorite all over Bangladesh. From various hotels to home parties, and especially during Eid-ul-Adha, this dish brings an extra shine to the dining table. The recipe is fairly simple, and the more time and care you invest, the richer the flavors will become. Here's how to make it:

Ingredients:

- **Beef:** 1 kg
- **Ginger paste:** 1 tablespoon
- **Garlic paste:** 1 tablespoon
- **Red Chili Powder:** 2 teaspoons
- **Turmeric powder:** 1 teaspoon
- **Cumin Powder:** 1 tablespoon
- **Coriander Powder:** 1 tablespoon
- **Garam masala powder:** 2 teaspoons
- **Fried Onion (Bereshta):** 1 cup
- **Onion, sliced:** 1/2 cup
- **Salt:** to taste
- **Plain yogurt:** 4 tablespoons
- **Bay leaves:** 3 pieces
- **Cinnamon stick:** 3 pieces
- **Green Cardamom:** 4 pieces
- **Star Anise:** 2 pieces
- **Black Cardamom:** 2 pieces
- **Cloves:** 5-6 pieces
- **Nutmeg powder:** 1/4 teaspoon
- **Mace powder:** 1/4 teaspoon
- **Radhuni Powder:** 1/2 teaspoon + 1/4 teaspoon
- **Black pepper powder:** 1 teaspoon
- **Roasted Cumin powder:** 1 teaspoon
- **Oil:** Fried onion oil 1/2 cup + Mustard Oil 1/2 cup (Total = 1 cup)

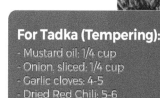

For Tadka (Tempering):

- Mustard oil: 1/4 cup
- Onion, sliced: 1/4 cup
- Garlic cloves: 4-5
- Dried Red Chili: 5-6
- Hot water: 1 Cup

Directions:

1. Start by marinating the beef with all the spices, yogurt, fried onions, and half of the oil. Allow it to sit for a couple of hours or overnight if possible for the flavors to meld.

2. In a heavy-bottomed pan, heat the remaining oil and add the beef mixture. Cook on medium flame till the meat starts to brown and the spices become fragrant.

3. Once the beef is browned and the spices are cooked, add hot water and allow the meat to simmer until it becomes tender and the water reduces, forming a thick gravy.

4. For the tadka, heat mustard oil in a separate pan, add sliced onions, garlic cloves, and dried red chili. Fry until the onions are golden.

5. Pour this tadka over the prepared beef and give it a good mix.

6. Serve hot with rice or parathas.

Note: For a genuine taste, it's recommended to use authentic spices native to Bangladesh.

3. Chittagong Traditional
Mejbani Chanar Dal *Recipe*

Introduction: Mejbani is an iconic cuisine from the southeastern region of Bangladesh, particularly in Chittagong. Traditionally, it refers to community feasts hosted by someone to resolve disputes, celebrate events, or simply for the love of food. While Mejbani is best known for its beef dishes, Chittagong's culinary repertoire boasts a variety of flavors, including those with lentils. The Chanar Dal (split chickpeas) recipe is a testament to this. Let's dive into this flavorful dish:

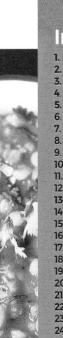

Ingredients:

1. Beef/Mutton with fat and bones - 600 grams
2. Split chickpeas (Chholar dal) - 1 cup
3. Mustard oil - 1/4 cup + 3 tablespoons
4. Chopped onions - 1 cup
5. Ginger paste - 1 tablespoon
6. Poppy seed paste - 1 teaspoon
7. Garlic paste - 1.5 teaspoons
8. Mustard paste - 1 tablespoon
9. Almond paste or Coconut paste - 1 tablespoon
10. Chili powder - 1 tablespoon
11. Turmeric powder - 1 teaspoon
12. Nutmeg and mace powder - 1/2 teaspoon
13. Cumin powder - 1 teaspoon
14. Coriander powder - 1 teaspoon
15. Garam masala powder - 1 teaspoon
16. Bay leaves - 3
17. Cinnamon - 2 sticks
18. Star anise - 2
19. Black pepper - 6
20. Cloves - 3
21. Black cardamom - 3
22. Green cardamom - 4
23. Green chilies - 10
24. Salt - to taste

Method:

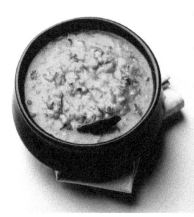

1. Soak the chickpeas in enough water. After 2 hours, drain the water, place the lentils in a pot, add 4 cups of water and some slit green chilies. Add 1 teaspoon of salt and cover. Wait until the lentils are 70% cooked. Once done, remove the green chilies with a spoon. Transfer the lentils to a bowl. Keep the lentils, chilies, and boiled water separately.

2. In a flat pan, add **1/4** cup of mustard oil. Once hot, add the chopped onions and whole garam masalas. Fry until golden brown. Then, add all the ground spices. Mix well, add the powdered spices and mix again. Add **1/4** cup of water, salt to taste, and previously boiled green chilies. Cover and cook for 5 minutes. Once the oil separates, add the beef or mutton. If there's more bone in the meat, it will taste better. Mix the meat well, cover the pan, and cook on low-medium heat for **10** minutes. Add enough water, cover, and cook the meat for **30-40** minutes. Stir occasionally. Once the meat is soft and tender, add the boiled chickpeas, mix, cover, and cook for **5** minutes. Then, add the reserved boiled water and continue to cook the meat on low-medium heat for 10 more minutes.

3. In another pan, heat 3 tablespoons of mustard oil. Once hot, add 1 teaspoon of the cooked lentil mixture. Fry a little and then add it to the pan with meat. Mix all the ingredients. Once it comes to a boil, remove from heat.

4. Chittagong Traditional Traditional

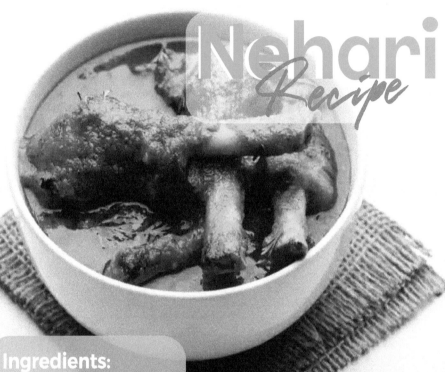

Ingredients:

Part 1:

- 4 beef trotters (Nala)
- 2 tablespoons ginger paste
- 2 tablespoons garlic paste
- 1 cup onion paste
- ½ cup almond paste
- 2 tablespoons white mustard seed paste
- 2 tablespoons poppy seed paste
- 1 tablespoon chili powder
- 2 tablespoons coriander powder
- 2 tablespoons cumin powder
- 2 tablespoons turmeric powder
- Garam masala and salt to taste

Part 2:

- 1 tablespoon garam masala powder
- 1 cup soybean oil
- 1 cup chopped onions
- 3 tablespoons chopped garlic

For sourness:

- Jujube, green mango, or tamarind to taste
- 10-12 green chilies
- 1 kg tomatoes

Instructions:

1. Prep the Trotters: Cut the beef trotters into pieces and wash them thoroughly. Combine with all the spices from Part 1 and marinate well.

2. Cook the Trotters: Place the marinated trotters in a pot, cover with water, and simmer for several hours until the meat is tender. Add more water as needed during cooking.

3. Add Sour Ingredients: Once the meat is tender, reduce the heat, and if the water level reduces, add more water. Then, add the ingredients for sourness, such as jujube, green mango, or tamarind, along with green chilies and tomatoes.

4. Prepare the Tempering: In a separate pan, heat the soybean oil from Part 2, and sauté the chopped onions and garlic until golden brown.

5. Combine and Simmer: Pour the onion and garlic oil mixture into the pot with the trotters. Add garam masala powder, cover, and simmer for another 10 to 15 minutes.

6. Serve: Remove from heat and serve hot with naan, roti, or rice.

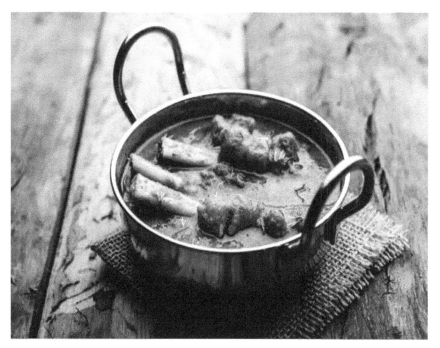

Note: To enhance the flavor of Nehari, consider using authentic, locally-produced spices.

The Chittagong culinary tradition is marked by its bold flavors and a blend of coastal ingredients. Whether it's the slow-cooked beef delicacy or the distinct flavor of dry fish, these recipes exemplify the richness and diversity of the region's food culture. Enjoying these dishes is not just a gastronomic delight but also a journey into the heart of Chittagong's cultural heritage.

Chapter 11:

My Culinary Journey

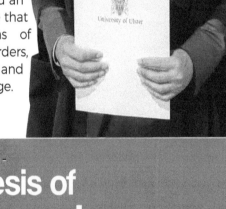

Every **individual's** culinary journey is unique, shaped by personal experiences, training, influences, and an inherent love for food. Mine is a tale that began in the bustling kitchens of Bangladesh and transcended borders, culminating in accolades and recognition on the international stage.

Section 11.1: Roots -
The Genesis of
My Culinary Journey

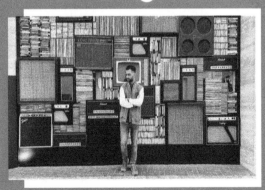

The heartbeat of my culinary journey commenced in the cozy confines of my family's kitchen in Bangladesh. Every early morning, as the sun began to cast its golden hue, I would be awakened by the inviting aroma of simmering curries, coupled with the rustle of freshly picked vegetables. These sensations were often punctuated by the melodic dance of spices being ground in the age-old mortar and pestle, each rhythm echoing the traditions of our ancestors.

My mother

, the maestro of our family kitchen, was my first guru. Under her watchful eyes, I learned not just recipes, but the very soul of Bangladeshi cuisine. She taught me that cooking was not just about mixing ingredients but about weaving stories, memories, and emotions into every dish. Each meal she pre pared was a tapestry of her love, dedication, and an embodiment of our cultural legacy. Her hands, seasoned with years of culinary experience, gracefully moved with purpose, molding me silently as I observed, learned, and imbibed.

As time moved on, other members of my family further enriched my culinary canvas. My grandmother, with her treasure trove of age-old recipes, introduced me to the ancestral wisdom of our cuisine. Each story she narrated, of her youth and the dishes she learned from her mother, added layers to my understanding. My uncles and aunts, each with their unique flair and specialties, expanded my horizons. From them, I learned the variations, the regional nuances, and the beautiful diversity that Bangladeshi cuisine had to offer.

These formative years, surrounded by a family deeply passionate about food, were the bedrock upon which my culinary dreams were built. Each lesson, each anecdote, and each shared meal, not only equipped me with skills but also instilled a deep sense of purpose and dedication to preserving and promoting our rich culinary heritage.

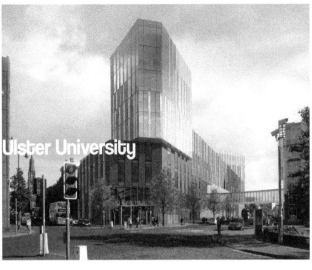

Section 11.2:
Education -
Mastering the Art at Ulster University

To refine my skills and gain a formal education in culinary arts, I decided to pursue an MSc degree from Ulster University in Belfast. This opportunity provided me with a comprehensive understanding of culinary science, global cuisines, and the delicate balance between tradition and innovation in food. Being part of the Super Star class of 2022 was an affirmation of my dedication and a stepping stone towards future successes.

Section 11.3:
Training -
Learning from the Masters

Post my academic pursuit, I was fortunate to work with culinary greats that shaped my skills and influenced my cooking style. I began my journey with **Michael Deane** in Northern Ireland, absorbing the fine nuances of British cuisine. Subsequently, I trained with the French culinary maestro, **Jean-Christophe Novelli**, where I immersed myself in the artistry of French cooking.

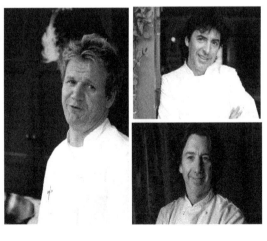

My journey continued under the mentorship of Gordon Ramsay, whose prowess in British cooking and work ethic left an indelible mark on me. Each of these experiences enriched my understanding of global cuisines and instilled a deep respect for the art of cooking.

Section 11.4:

Leadership in Cuisine:
Mentoring 100,000+ Global Talents.

My journey, deeply influenced by the teachings of culinary legends, equipped me with a profound spectrum of culinary knowledge and a deep-seated reverence for the art. Rather than confining my expertise to a single kitchen, I chose to embrace a wider calling. Today, as a dedicated mentor, chef, and teacher, I've imparted my wisdom to over 100,000 students globally. And the legacy continues to flourish as that number grows daily, showcasing an ever-expanding commitment to fostering the next generation of culinary talent.

Section 11.5:

Culinary Bootcamp &
Diverse Courses:

At the helm of the culinary world, I realized the importance of disseminating knowledge and decided to spearhead a comprehensive culinary bootcamp. This initiative offers an array of courses, ranging from foundational to advanced, encompassing a myriad of culinary techniques, world cuisines, and dietary considerations. Each course is meticulously designed to provide participants with a profound understanding and hands-on experience, enabling them to hone their skills and develop a distinct culinary identity.

Leadership & Digital Impact
in the Culinary World:

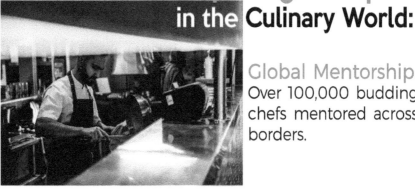

Global Mentorship:
Over 100,000 budding chefs mentored across borders.

Digital Engagement: Actively nurturing culinary enthusiasts via Facebook and YouTube with insightful videos, recipes, and live interactions.

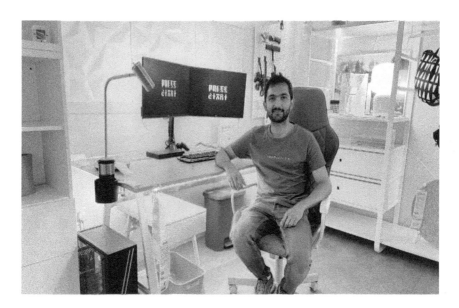

From Bangladesh to Global Stardom:
Established as a restaurateur, author, and mentor, I proudly stand as the top chef both in Bangladesh and the UK, and crowned as the 1st Level 7 chef in Bangladesh.

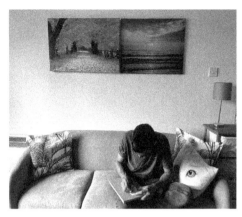

Legacy & Inspiration:

While celebrating international acclaim, my heart remains tethered to promoting Bangladeshi cuisine with unmatched passion. My trajectory, from Bangladesh's home kitchens to global recognition, stands as an emblem of passion, perseverance, and continuous growth, aiming to inspire others to delve deep into the culinary treasures of Bangladesh.

Digital Engagement & Social Media Presence:

In this interconnected era, the digital realm is a powerful platform to connect, share, and learn. I actively engage with culinary enthusiasts on Facebook and YouTube, sharing enlightening cooking videos, recipes, and live sessions. These platforms serve as interactive spaces where budding chefs can ask questions, seek advice, and receive real-time feedback, creating a global community of culinary aficionados.

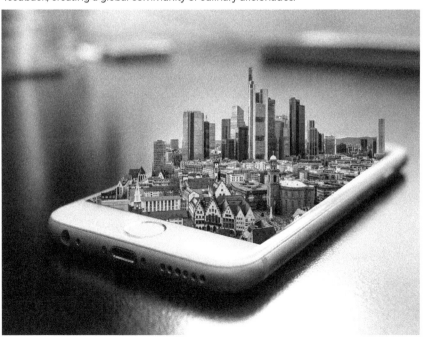

Chapter 12: The Future of Bangladeshi Cuisine

Bangladeshi cuisine, with its rich flavors and deep-seated tradition, is a culinary gem that is steadily gaining recognition on the global stage. As we look to the future, it is important to consider the role this cuisine can play in the global culinary landscape and the steps we need to take to preserve its authenticity while allowing it to evolve.

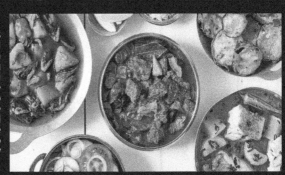

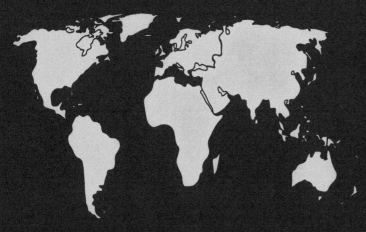

Global Influence

Bangladeshi cuisine's global influence has been on an impressive rise, making its presence felt far beyond the nation's borders. This growth can be attributed to several key factors:

1. International
Chefs and Restaurateurs:

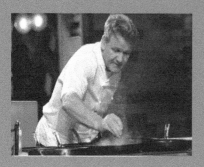

Explanation: Bangladeshi chefs and restaurateurs working internationally are ambassadors of their culinary heritage. By incorporating traditional Bangladeshi techniques and flavors into global kitchens, they have brought a taste of Bangladesh to the world.

Impact: Heightened curiosity and demand for Bangladeshi dishes.

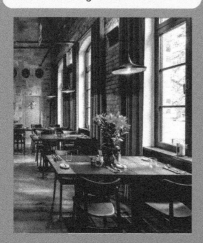

2. Cultural Festivals
and Food Fairs:

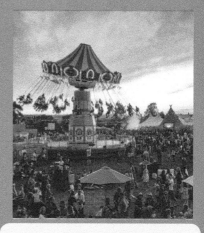

Explanation: Participation in international food festivals and cultural fairs showcases Bangladeshi cuisine to a wider audience. Such platforms allow people to experience the rich flavors and textures that define Bangladeshi food.

Impact: Builds cultural bridges and encourages culinary tourism.

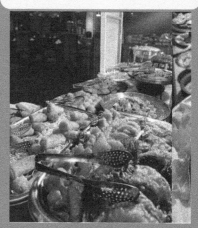

3. Global Media
Exposure:

Explanation: Features in international culinary magazines, TV shows, and documentaries have contributed to a growing interest in Bangladeshi food. Social media, food blogs, and online platforms also play a role in making the cuisine accessible to a global audience.

Impact: Broadens awareness and educates people about the uniqueness of the cuisine.

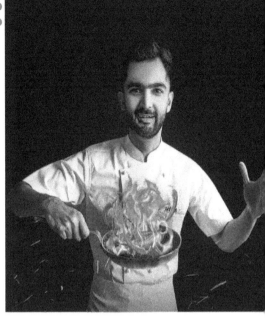

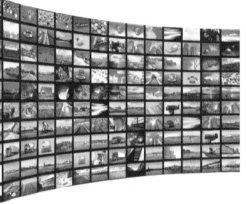

4. Migration and Diaspora Communities:

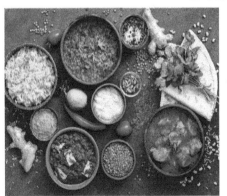

Explanation: Bangladeshi communities living abroad often set up restaurants and food businesses that cater to their local tastes and to others interested in trying something new. This makes Bangladeshi cuisine available in many parts of the world.

Impact: Reinforces the presence of Bangladeshi food culture and opens it to new audiences.

5. Collaboration with Renowned
Global Brands:

Explanation: Collaborations between Bangladeshi chefs and renowned global culinary brands, hotels, and restaurants give credibility and status to Bangladeshi cuisine.

Impact: Places Bangladeshi cuisine on a pedestal with other respected culinary traditions.

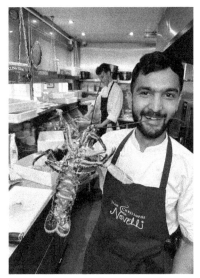

6. Educational
Institutions:

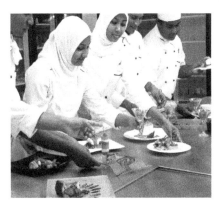

Explanation: Culinary schools embracing Bangladeshi cooking techniques and including them in their curriculum provide an opportunity for the next generation of chefs to learn and innovate with these traditions.

Impact: Ensures the continuity and evolution of Bangladeshi cuisine in modern gastronomy.

7. The Chef Model Design:
Arfatul Islam

1. Foundation Skills
- **Culinary Techniques:** Knife skills, sautéing, baking, grilling, etc.
- **Basic Cooking Methods:** Boiling, steaming, frying, roasting, etc.
- **Safety & Hygiene:** Safe food handling, proper cleaning, and sanitation practices.
- **Ingredient Knowledge:** Understanding different ingredients, their properties, and how they interact.

2. Culinary Knowledge
- **World Cuisines:** Study major world cuisines, from French to Chinese, Indian to Mediterranean.
- **Dietary Requirements:** Vegan, gluten-free, allergies, religious diets, etc.
- **Food Science:** Understand the chemistry and physics behind cooking.
- **Nutrition:** Knowledge of the health aspects of ingredients and meals.

3. Innovation & Creativity
- **Recipe Development:** Creating and refining original recipes.
- **Presentation:** Developing plate design and presentation skills.
- **Taste Balance:** Understanding flavor profiles and balancing sweet, sour, salty, bitter, and umami.

4. Business Acumen
- **Kitchen Management:** Inventory, staffing, equipment maintenance.
- **Financial Skills:** Budgeting, cost analysis, profit margins.
- **Marketing & Branding:** Building a personal brand or restaurant brand.
- **Customer Service:** Ensuring customer satisfaction, handling feedback.

5. Interpersonal Skills
- **Team Leadership:** Leading a kitchen team efficiently.
- **Communication:** Clear instructions, active listening, feedback reception.
- **Conflict Resolution:** Managing disagreements in the kitchen environment.
- **Mentorship:** Guiding younger chefs and kitchen staff.

6. Continuous Learning
- **Workshops & Courses:** Regularly update skills with advanced courses.
- **Networking:** Join chef associations, attend culinary events.
- **Reading & Research:** Stay updated with culinary trends, new ingredients, and techniques.
- **Feedback Reception:** Always be open to feedback and criticism.

7. Self-care & Well-being
- **Physical Fitness:** Maintain stamina and strength for long kitchen hours.
- **Mental Health:** Stress management, work-life balance.
- **Passion & Motivation:** Continually reignite passion for cooking and creativity.

8. Environmental & Ethical Responsibility
- **Sustainable Cooking:** Usage of local and seasonal ingredients, reducing waste.
- **Ethical Sourcing:** Ensure ingredients are ethically sourced, promoting fair trade.
- **Community Engagement:** Participate in community services, offer culinary training.

9. Digital Era Adaptability
- **Online Presence:** Active profiles on social media, sharing recipes, and cooking videos.
- **Tech-savviness:** Understanding kitchen tech, apps, reservation software, etc.
- **Online Learning:** Utilizing online platforms for culinary courses, webinars, etc.

10. Final Ingredient - Passion & Persistence
- Dedication: Being dedicated to the art and craft of cooking.
- Love for Food: The inherent love for food and the joy it brings to people.
- Persistence: Facing challenges, failures, and still pushing through with determination.

The Chef Model Design: Pathway to Culinary Excellence emphasizes mastering foundational culinary techniques, gaining comprehensive knowledge of global cuisines, and fostering innovation. It underscores the importance of business savvy in kitchen management and branding while enhancing interpersonal skills for effective team leadership. The model champions continuous learning, ensuring adaptability in the digital era, and underlines the significance of self-care, ethical responsibility, and sustainability. At its core, it celebrates the unwavering dedication, love for food, and resilience intrinsic to the culinary journey.

Section 12.2: Opportunities and Challenges

While the global exposure presents opportunities for Bangladeshi cuisine, it also brings challenges. The opportunity lies in elevating Bangladeshi cuisine to the level of other well-recognized global cuisines and leveraging this recognition to promote tourism and cultural exchange. The challenge, however, is to ensure that as the cuisine gains global popularity, its authenticity is preserved, and it does not lose its unique identity.Certainly! Here's a more detailed exploration of the opportunities and challenges in Section 12.2:

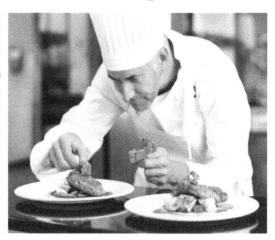

Opportunities

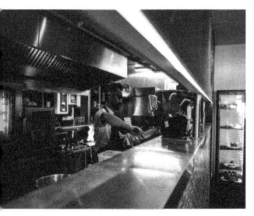

1. Global Recognition:

Description: Achieving global recognition can elevate Bangladeshi cuisine to the level of other wellknown culinary traditions.

Methods: Collaborating with world-renowned chefs, participating in international food festivals, and utilizing media exposure.

Impact: Increases tourism, fosters cultural understanding, and boosts national pride.

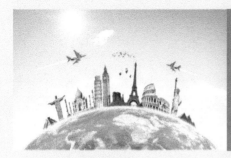

2. Tourism Boost:

Description: By promoting the country's rich culinary heritage, Bangladesh can attract food enthusiasts from around the world.

Methods: Creating culinary tours, hosting food festivals, and advertising through travel agencies.

Impact: Economic growth and increased interest in Bangladeshi culture.

3. Culinary Innovation:

Description: Fusion of traditional Bangladeshi flavors with modern culinary techniques can lead to unique and innovative dishes.

Methods: Collaborate with culinary schools, experiment with contemporary techniques, and encourage innovation in local restaurants.

Impact: Positions Bangladeshi cuisine as a creative and evolving tradition.

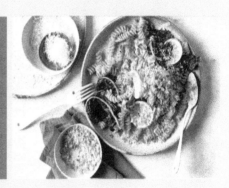

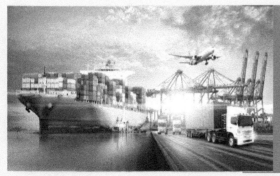

4. Export Opportunities:

Description: Popularizing Bangladeshi dishes may lead to increased demand for specific indigenous ingredients abroad.

Methods: Build connections with international suppliers and retailers.

Impact: Opens new markets for Bangladeshi agricultural products.

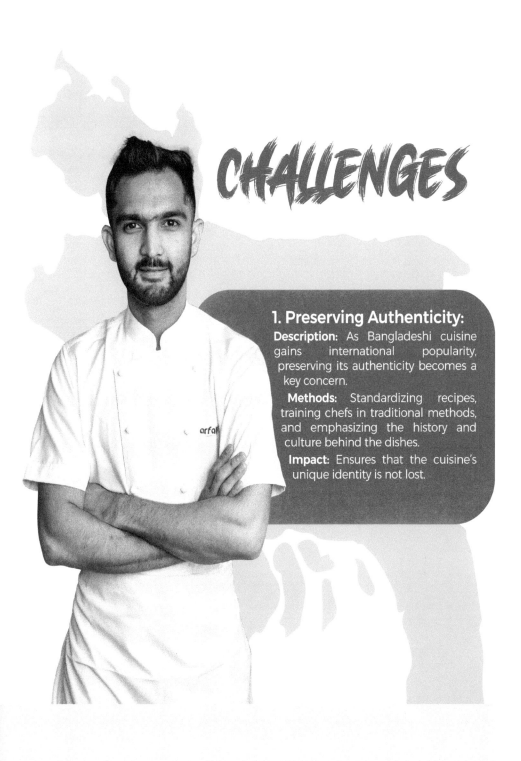

CHALLENGES

1. Preserving Authenticity:

Description: As Bangladeshi cuisine gains international popularity, preserving its authenticity becomes a key concern.

Methods: Standardizing recipes, training chefs in traditional methods, and emphasizing the history and culture behind the dishes.

Impact: Ensures that the cuisine's unique identity is not lost.

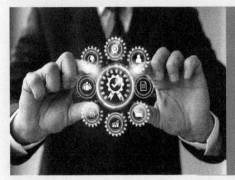

2. Quality Control:

Description: Maintaining consistent quality across various platforms and locations is vital to build trust and reputation.

Methods: Implementing quality assurance processes, continuous training, and sourcing quality ingredients.

Impact: Builds trust and maintains the high standards of the cuisine.

3. Accessibility of Ingredients:

Description: Ensuring the availability of specific Bangladeshi ingredients in foreign markets may be challenging.

Methods: Collaborate with global suppliers and explore substitutions that do not compromise authenticity.

Impact: Helps in making Bangladeshi cuisine more approachable globally.

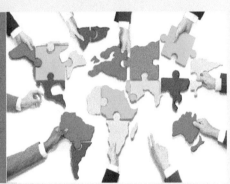

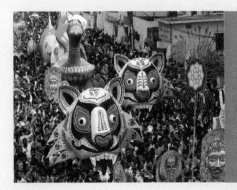

4. Cultural Sensitivity:

Description: Adapting Bangladeshi cuisine to different cultures without offending local sensibilities.

Methods: Understanding cultural norms, preferences, and taboos in target markets.

Impact: Facilitates smoother acceptance and integration of Bangladeshi cuisine worldwide.

Section 12.3:
Embracing Innovation

The future of Bangladeshi cuisine lies in the balance of tradition and innovation. While preserving traditional recipes and cooking methods, it is also crucial to experiment and innovate. This may involve incorporating modern cooking techniques, presenting dishes in new ways, or adapting recipes to cater to global dietary trends without losing the essence of Bangladeshi flavors.

Section 12.4:
Sustainability in the Culinary Practice

Sustainability is a global concern that also applies to the culinary world. For the future of Bangladeshi cuisine, it will be important to ensure that cooking practices are environmentally sustainable. This may involve promoting the use of locally sourced ingredients, reducing food waste, and raising awareness about sustainable eating practices.

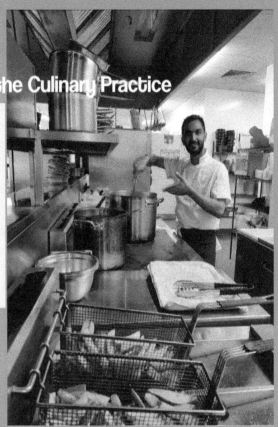

Section 12.5:
Culinary Education and Mentorship

For Bangladeshi cuisine to thrive in the future, the next generation of chefs needs to be trained and mentored effectively. It is important to pass on the knowledge of traditional cooking methods while also teaching modern culinary skills.

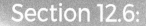

Section 12.6:

My Vision by
Arfatul Islam

My vision is clear:

to elevate Bangladeshi cuisine to Michelin star acclaim, making it more than just an exotic flavor. It's a representation of our rich heritage, passion, and traditions. Through this book, I aim to inspire readers to delve deep into our culinary legacy, merging age-old recipes with contemporary methods.By sharing this journey, I hope to connect our past with the present, turning every dish into a global ambassador for Bangladesh. Let's work collectively to ensure Bangladeshi flavors echo in food enthusiasts' hearts across the globe. Dive into this culinary adventure and relish the essence of Bangladesh with every bite.

Bangladeshi cuisine and bring it global recognition, here are some concrete steps and points that canhelp guide the journey:

1. Culinary Schooling and Training:

Partner with international culinary schools to offer courses specializing in Bangladeshi cuisine. This provides legitimacy and promotes knowledge exchange.

2. Global Bangladeshi Food Festivals:

Organize and participate in food festivals across major cities worldwide. Use them as platforms to showcase traditional and fusion dishes.

3. Collaborations:

Work with internationally recognized chefs to blend their expertise with Bangladeshi flavors, thereby creating unique fusion dishes.

4. Documentary and Media Promotion:

Partner with streaming platforms like Netflix or Amazon Prime to produce documentaries or shows that delve deep into the culinary heritage of Bangladesh.

5. Pop-up Restaurants:

Establish temporary restaurants in major world cities. This can generate buzz and offer a taste of Bangladeshi cuisine to a wider audience.

6. Innovate and Modernize:

While staying true to roots, experiment with modern culinary techniques (like molecular gastronomy) to give traditional dishes a contemporary twist.

7. Ingredient Accessibility:

Collaborate with suppliers and exporters to make Bangladeshi ingredients available worldwide. This helps chefs and enthusiasts replicate the dishes authentically.

8. Sustainable and Ethical Practices:

Emphasize the use of local, organic, and sustainably sourced ingredients in recipes. This resonates with global trends towards ethical eating.

9. Michelin Guide Focus:

Study the criteria Michelin inspectors use to judge restaurants. Ensure Bangladeshi restaurants meet and exceed these standards.

10. Culinary Tours:

Organize guided tours in Bangladesh for food enthusiasts and critics. This immersive experience can serve as a deep dive into the food culture.

11. Digital Presence:

Create a strong online presence through blogs, YouTube cooking series, and social media campaigns that narrate the stories behind each dish.

12. Workshops and Masterclasses:

Offer masterclasses in major cities around the world, educating people about the techniques, flavors, and history of Bangladeshi cuisine.

13. Networking:

Build relationships with global culinary influencers, food critics, and journalists. Their endorsements can significantly elevate the cuisine's profile.

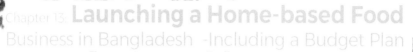

Chapter 13: Launching a Home-based Food Business in Bangladesh -Including a Budget Plan

Venturing into the world of food entrepreneurship can be both challenging and rewarding. For aspiring culinary entrepreneurs in Bangladesh, this chapter will guide you on how to build a successful career by starting a food business at home. A critical aspect of this process is planning your budget efficiently.

Section 13.1: Setting the Foundation

1. Market Research: Dedicate at least 3 weeks for comprehensive research. Understand regional preferences and the popularity of different cuisines.

2. Trend Analysis: Review at least five years of food industry data to predict upcoming trends.

3. Competitor Assessment: Identify top 5-7 direct competitors. Understand their strengths and weaknesses through customer reviews and personal assessments.

Section 13.2: Crafting a Business Plan

1. Concept Elaboration: Define your niche and differentiate from competitors.

2. Financial Forecasts: Project financials for 1, 3, and 5 years.

3. SWOT Analysis: Identify strengths, weaknesses, opportunities, and threats.

Section 13.3: Budget Planning

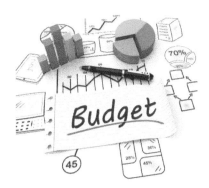

1. Startup Costs: Allot at least 20% more than your initial calculations for unforeseen expenses during the setup.

2. Operating Costs: Analyze monthly expenditures for the first three months to get an accurate picture.

3. Contingency Funds: Set aside at least 10% of your monthly operating costs for unplanned expenses.

Section 13.4: Legalities and Registrations

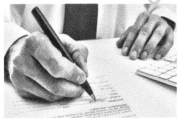

1. Licenses: Factor in costs for at least 3-5 different licenses depending on local regulations.

2. Food Safety Compliance: Budget for regular audits and certifications.

3. Tax Consultation: A dedicated portion for tax consultation to prevent any legal issues down the road.

Section 13.5: Setting Up Your Kitchen

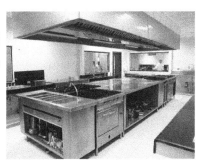

1. Space Analysis: Ensure at least 60% of your kitchen space is devoted to cooking and prep, with 40% left for storage and cleaning.

2. Equipment Audit: Monthly checks to account for wear and tear, ensuring consistency in food quality.

3. Safety Standards: Allocate funds for fire extinguishers, first aid kits, and other safety essentials.

Section 13.6: Sourcing Ingredients

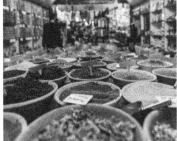

1. Vendor Contracts: Negotiate terms with at least 3 main vendors. Secure discounts for bulk purchases.

2. Quality Checks: Allocate resources for weekly quality checks.

3. Seasonal Ingredients: Plan for price variations due to seasonal availability.

Section 13.7: Marketing Your Business

1. Digital Presence: Dedicate 40% of your marketing budget to develop and maintain a robust online presence.

2. Local Campaigns: Engage in at least two local events monthly for direct engagement.

3. Feedback Mechanisms: Implement at least two platforms or methods for customers to share feedback

Section 13.8:
Scaling Your Business

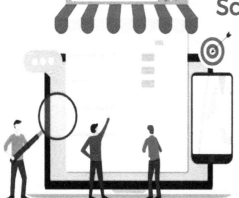

ics: Set tangible milestones like achieving 'x' number of ount of profits.

lysis: For physical expansion, iree possible locations based emographics and footfall.

Planning: Have a plan for ional capital, be it through or selffunding.

Section 13.9:
Staffing and Training

While you might start solo, as the business grows, hiring help becomes essential. This section focuses on the costs associated with:

1. Recruitment: Posting job ads, conducting interviews, and potential hiring agency fees.

2. Salaries: Wages for chefs, helpers, delivery personnel, and administrative staff.

3. Training: To maintain consistent quality, periodic training sessions for your staff are crucial. This can include culinary training, customer service lessons, and health and safety guidelines.

4. Employee Benefits: Health insurance, paid leaves, and other perks.

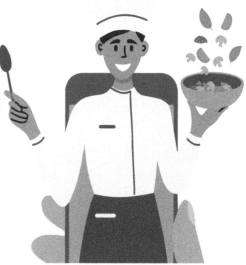

169

Section 13.10:
Customer Engagement and Feedback

Building a loyal customer base is critical. This section involves:

1. Loyalty Programs: Costs associated with setting up reward systems, discounts, or loyalty cards.
2. Feedback Platforms: Invest in platforms where customers can leave reviews and provide constructive feedback.
3. Customer Service: Budget for hiring customer service representatives or chat support, especially if you're going online.

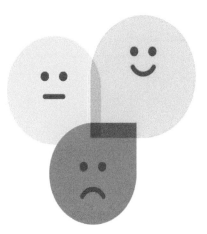

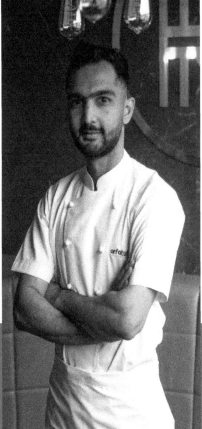

Section 13.11:
Continuous Improvement

The culinary world is always evolving, and staying stagnant can be detrimental:

1. Research and Development: Periodically test new recipes or tweak existing ones based on feedback.
2. Skill Upgradation: Attend culinary workshops, courses, or food expos to keep up with industry standards and trends.
3. Equipment Upgradation: As technology advances, consider upgrading equipment to improve efficiency.

Section 13.12: **Risk Management**

Every business faces risks, and mitigating them is crucial:

1. Insurance: Opt for coverage against potential risks, such as property damage, theft, or liability claims.
2. Health and Safety: Regular audits of kitchen safety standards to prevent mishaps.
3. Financial Audits: Periodic checks to ensure all transactions are transparent, and there's no discrepancy in accounts.

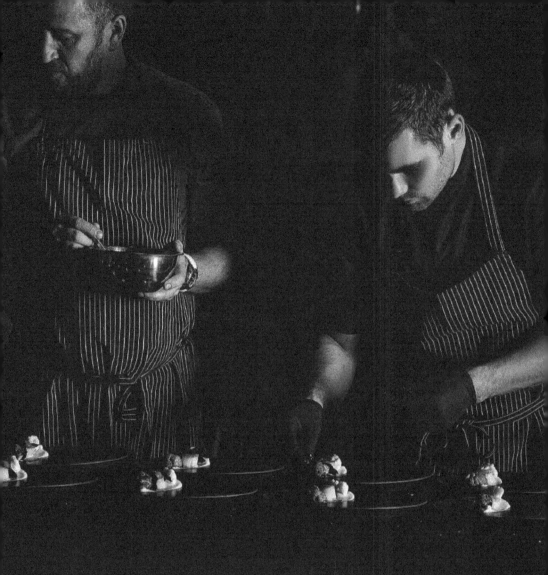

By meticulously *planning* each aspect of your culinary venture, you're not just ensuring smooth operations but also preparing your business for sustainable growth. With dedication, hard work, and careful planning, success will undoubtedly be on the menu.

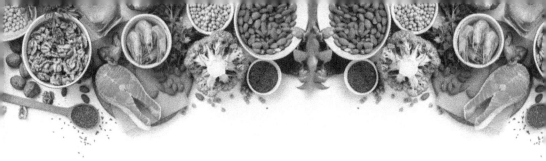

Chapter 14: The Panorama of Possibilities:
Every Flavor, Every Tale

Bangladeshi Cuisine: A Balance of Tradition and Nutrition – 7 Day Healthy Diet Plan

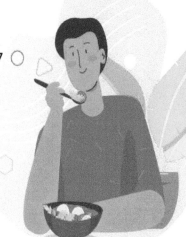

Creating a balanced diet chart involves considering an individual's daily caloric needs, their level of physical activity, any specific dietary restrictions, and their personal food preferences. That being said, I can provide you with a general diet chart based on healthy Bangladeshi food options. Here's a 7-day plan that you can modify to suit your needs:

Day 1:

- **Breakfast:** Chola Bhuna (spicy chickpeas) with whole wheat roti.

- **Mid-morning snack:** Fresh guava.

- **Lunch:** Mixed vegetable curry with brown rice, a side of dhal and cucumber salad.

- **Afternoon snack:** A handful of mixed nuts.

- **Dinner:** Grilled fish with stir-fried vegetables.

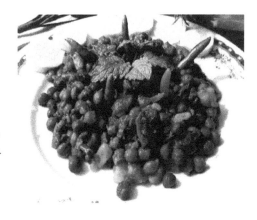

Day 2:

- **Breakfast:** Vegetable Upma made with semolina.
- **Mid-morning snack:** A banana.
- **Lunch:** Chicken curry with brown rice, side of mixed vegetable bharta.
- **Afternoon snack:** A cup of yogurt.
- **Dinner:** Khichuri (rice and lentil porridge) with a side of mixed pickles.

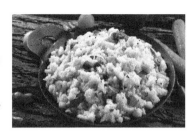

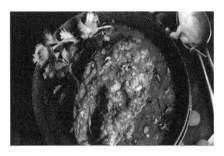

Day 3:

- **Breakfast:** Dalia (broken wheat porridge) with mixedfruits.
- **Mid-morning snack:** A handful of grapes.
- **Lunch:** Fish curry with brown rice, side of spinach bhaji.
- **Afternoon snack:** Sliced cucumber and carrots.
- **Dinner:** Chicken stew with whole wheat roti.

Day 4:

- **Breakfast:** Egg bhurji (scrambled eggs) with whole wheat bread.
- **Mid-morning snack:** An apple.
- **Lunch:** Shorshe Ilish (Hilsa in mustard sauce) with
  brown rice, side of mixed vegetable bhaji.
- **Afternoon snack:** A bowl of yogurt with sliced mango.
- **Dinner:** Vegetable pulao with raita.

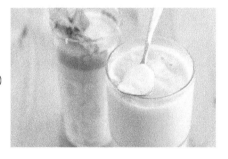

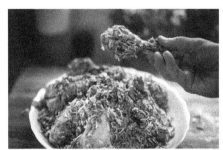

Day 5:

- **Breakfast:** Paratha with aloo bhaji (potato curry).
- **Mid-morning snack:** Orange.
- **Lunch:** Chicken biryani with a side of mixed vegetable salad.
- **Afternoon snack:** A handful of mixed nuts.
- **Dinner:** Grilled fish with stir-fried vegetables.

173

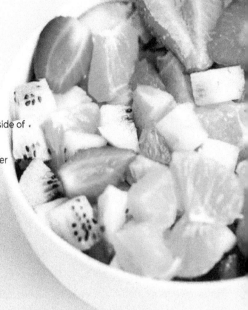

Day 6:

- **Breakfast:** Vegetable stuffed whole wheat roti with a side of yogurt.
- **Mid-morning snack:** A banana.
- **Lunch:** Dal with brown rice, brinjal bhaji, and cucumber salad.
- **Afternoon snack:** A bowl of mixed fruit.
- **Dinner:** Mutton curry with whole wheat roti.

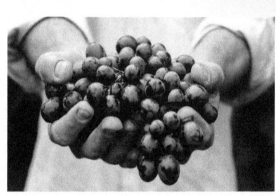

Day 7:

- **Breakfast:** Poha (flattened rice) with mixed vegetables.
- **Mid-morning snack:** A handful of grapes.
- **Lunch:** Fish curry with brown rice, side of mixed vegetable bharta.
- **Afternoon snack:** Sliced cucumber and carrots.
- **Dinner:** Chicken stew with whole wheat roti.

Remember to drink plenty of water throughout the day and try to include a daily exercise routine in your lifestyle for better health. This chart is quite general and might need adjustments according to your specific nutritional needs. Please consult with a nutritionist or a healthcare provider for a personalized meal plan.

Creating a healthy and balanced diet plan requires an understanding of an individual's daily calorie needs, health conditions, physical activity level, age, and sex. However, I can give you a general idea of a balanced diet plan featuring Bangladeshi foods. Always consult with a healthcare provider or a registered dietitian to personalize a meal plan for your unique needs.

One-day balanced Diet plan with traditional Bangladeshi foods:

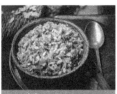

Breakfast:
- Bowl of 'Chire Bhaja' (Fried Flattened Rice) with Peanuts and Raisins.
- A Banana or a small Mango.

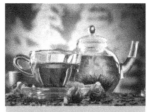

Mid-Morning Snack:
- A cup of green tea with a handful of mixed nuts (avoid salted or sweetened versions).

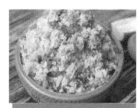

Lunch:
- A portion of 'Bhuna Khichuri' (a dish made from rice and lentils) with a side of mixed vegetable curry.
- A small bowl of 'Doi' (Yogurt) to aid digestion.

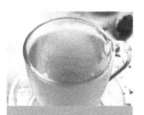

Afternoon Snack:
- A cup of 'Cha' (tea) without sugar.
- A small bowl of 'Muri' (puffed rice) with chopped cucumber, tomato, and a squeeze of lemon.

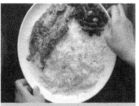

Dinner:
- A portion of 'Fish Curry' with 'Bhat' (Boiled Rice).
- A side of 'Shobji' (Sauteed or steamed seasonal vegetables).

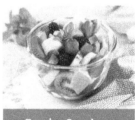

Evening Snack:
- A bowl of mixed fruits.

Note: Remember to adjust the portion sizes according to your personal dietary needs and goals. Also, try to include a variety of vegetables in your meals and rotate your protein sources **(like fish, lentils, c hicken,** etc.) throughout the week to ensure a wide spectrum of nutrients. It's also important to drink plenty of water throughout the day.

Remember, the key to a healthy diet is balance, moderation, and variety. Enjoy your culinary journey to a healthier you!

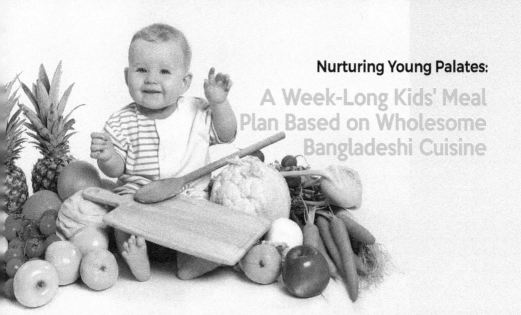

Nurturing Young Palates:
A Week-Long Kids' Meal Plan Based on Wholesome Bangladeshi Cuisine

Day 1:
- **Breakfast:** Wheat Roti with Egg Omelet
- **Lunch:** Chicken Pulao with Cucumber Salad
- **Snack:** Fresh Mango Slices
- **Dinner:** Fish Curry with Steamed Rice and Sauteed Spinach

Day 2:
- **Breakfast:** Vegetable Upma (Savory Semolina Porridge)
- **Lunch:** Lentil Soup with Rice and Carrot sticks
- **Snack:** Banana and Yogurt Smoothie
- **Dinner:** Chicken and Vegetable Stir Fry with Chapati

Day 3:
- **Breakfast:** Pancakes with Honey and Fresh Fruits
- **Lunch:** Beef Biryani with Raita (Yogurt Salad)
- **Snack:** Mixed Nuts and Raisins
- **Dinner:** Mashed Potatoes with Grilled Fish and Steamed Vegetables

Day 4:
- **Breakfast:** Cheese Sandwich with Fresh Orange Juice
- **Lunch:** Chicken Korma with Jeera Rice
- **Snack:** Apple and Peanut Butter
- **Dinner:** Vegetable Khichuri (Rice and Lentils) with Yogurt

Day 5:
- **Breakfast:** Vegetable Stuffed Paratha with Fresh Lassi (Yogurt Drink)
- **Lunch:** Shrimp Curry with Rice and Mixed Vegetable Salad
- **Snack:** Freshly Cut Papaya
- **Dinner:** Egg Curry with Roti and Cucumber Salad

Day 6:
- **Breakfast:** Poha (Flattened Rice) with Fresh Fruits
- **Lunch:** Mutton Pulao with Raita (Yogurt Salad)
- **Snack:** Grilled Cheese Sandwich
- **Dinner:** Mixed Vegetable Curry with Rice

Day 7:
- **Breakfast:** Scrambled Eggs with Toast and Freshly Squeezed Orange Juice
- **Lunch:** Fish Biryani with Salad
- **Snack:** Fresh Mango Lassi (Yogurt Drink)
- **Dinner:** Chana Dal (Split Chickpeas) with Roti and Mixed Vegetables

Please note: Portion sizes should be suitable for children's needs and dietary restrictions should be considered. As children's nutritional needs vary, it's advisable to consult with a pediatrician or nutritionist when significantly altering a child's diet.

Growing Up with Flavors of Bangladesh:

A Wholesome and Kid-friendly Meal Plan

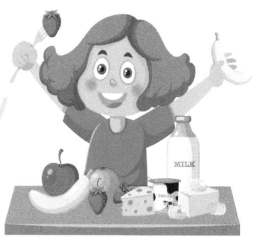

Breakfast:

Ruti (Flatbread): A staple breakfast item in Bangladesh, made with whole wheat flour, which is rich in fiber and aids digestion.

Egg Bhurji: Scrambled eggs with finely chopped onions, tomatoes, and a sprinkle of turmeric and cumin powder. It's a great source of protein for kids.

Milk: A glass of warm milk with a bit of honey for sweetness. It's rich in calcium and helps in the growth and development of strong bones and teeth.

Mid-Morning Snack:

Fruit Chaat: A simple and refreshing fruit salad made with seasonal fruits such as mangoes, bananas, and apples. This can be sprinkled with a dash of chaat masala to enhance the taste.

Lunch:

Khichuri (Rice and Lentils): A wholesome, one-pot dish made with rice, lentils, vegetables, and mild spices. This dish is well-balanced and packed with proteins, carbs, and vitamins.

Chicken Roast: A lightly spiced, roasted chicken dish that's popular in Bangladeshi cuisine and a good source of protein.

Mixed Vegetable Curry: A light curry made with seasonal vegetables, cooked with mild spices. It is a good source of various nutrients.

Afternoon Snack:

Muri (Puffed Rice): This can be served with a side of chana (chickpeas) or peanuts for added protein.

Dinner:

Fish Curry with Rice: Fish is a big part of Bangladeshi cuisine and is a good source of Omega-3 fatty acids. This can be served with a side of white rice, which is a staple in Bangladeshi households.

pinach Bhaji: A simple stir fry made with spinach. It's a great source of iron and vitamins.

Evening Snack (before bed):

Mishti Doi (Sweet Yogurt): This dessert is not only a favorite among children but is also a good source of probiotics, helping in digestion.

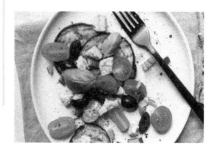

Remember to adjust portion sizes according to the age and activity level of your child. The aim is to give them a balanced diet that includes a variety of nutrients essential for their growth and development.

Sustaining Wellness with Bangladeshi Flavors:
A Diabetes-Friendly Meal Plan

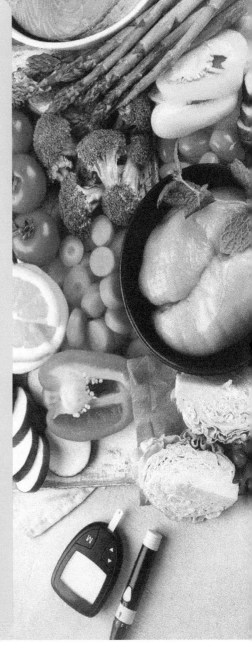

Breakfast:

Whole Wheat Paratha: This flatbread made with whole wheat flour is rich in fiber and has a lower glycemic index, making it suitable for a diabetic diet.

Egg Bhurji: Scrambled eggs with finely chopped onions, tomatoes, and a sprinkle of turmeric and cumin. Eggs are a great source of protein and will help keep you feeling full.

Cucumber and Tomato Salad: This fresh salad is low in carbs and high in fiber.

Mid-Morning Snack:

A handful of Nuts: Almonds, walnuts, or any other nut of choice. They are high in fiber and healthy fats, which are beneficial for blood sugar control

Lunch:

Brown Rice Khichuri (Rice and Lentils): A wholesome dish made with brown rice, lentils, and vegetables, spiced mildly. Brown rice is high in fiber and helps control blood sugar levels.

Grilled Fish: High in protein and omega-3 fatty acids, grilled fish is a healthy choice.

Spinach Bhaji: A simple stir fry made with spinach, a great source of iron and fiber.

Afternoon Snack:

Mixed Berries: A cup of mixed berries can be a sweet yet low-glycemic index treat.

Dinner:

Quinoa Pulao with Vegetables: Quinoa is a great substitute for rice in a diabetic diet, and it is high in protein and fiber.

Chicken Curry: Made with skinless chicken and a variety of spices, this dish is high in protein.

Mixed Vegetable Curry: A curry made with seasonal vegetables, providing a variety of vitamins and minerals.

Evening Snack (before bed):

Greek Yogurt with a sprinkle of flaxseeds: Greek yogurt is low in carbs and high in protein, and flaxseeds are rich in fiber and omega-3 fatty acids.

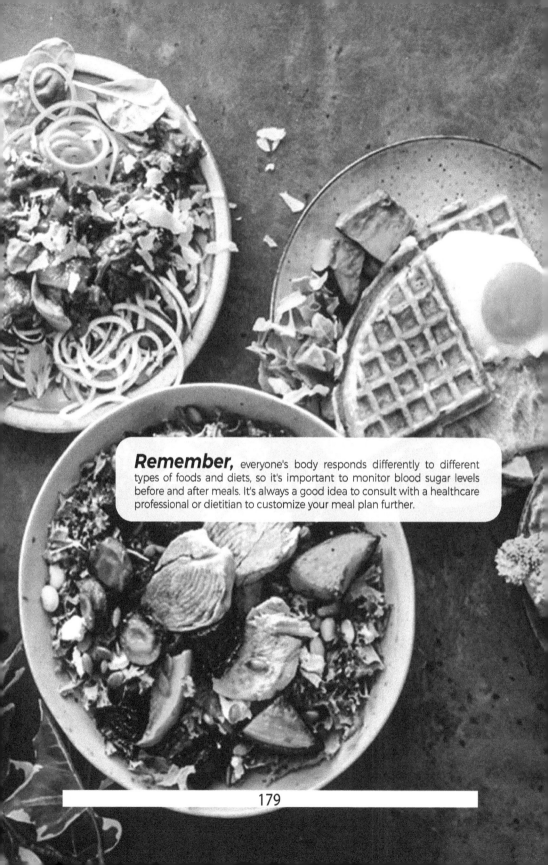

Remember, everyone's body responds differently to different types of foods and diets, so it's important to monitor blood sugar levels before and after meals. It's always a good idea to consult with a healthcare professional or dietitian to customize your meal plan further.

Heart-Healthy Bangladeshi Feast:
A Cholesterol-Friendly Meal Plan

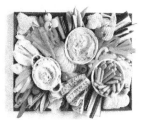

Breakfast:

Chola Bhuna (Chickpea Stir-Fry): A fiber-rich and heart-healthy breakfast, made with boiled chickpeas stirfried with tomatoes, onions, and minimal oil.

Whole Wheat Roti: A high-fiber, low- fat alternative to traditional flatbreads.

Mid-Morning Snack:

Mixed Berries: A handful of mixed berries are a great source of antioxidants and fiber, which can help lower cholesterol levels.

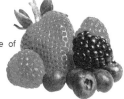

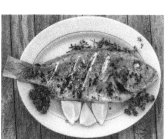

Lunch:

Brown Rice: A fiber-rich alternative to white rice that can help lower cholesterol.

Masoor Dal (Red Lentil Soup): Lentils are packed with protein and fiber, making them beneficial for heart health.

Bhindi Bhaji (Okra Stir Fry): Okra is known for its high fiber content and its ability to help lower cholesterol.

Afternoon Snack:

Carrot and Cucumber Sticks with Hummus: Raw vegetables are a great source of fiber and hummus provides healthy fats.

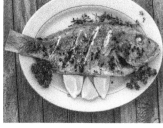

Dinner:

Grilled Fish with Lemon and Turmeric: Fish is high in omega-3 fatty acids, which are good for heart health.

Mixed Vegetable Curry: This curry is full of various vitamins and minerals, and high in fiber.

Quinoa: A protein-packed grain that is also high in fiber.

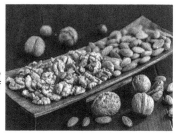

Evening Snack (before bed):

Almonds and Walnuts: Both these nuts are known to be good for heart health due to their high content of monounsaturated fats and fiber.

Please note, this meal plan is designed to help you control your cholesterol levels, but everyone is unique and responses to diets can vary . Therefore, you should always check with a healthcare professional or dietitian to tailor a meal plan that best fits your personal needs and conditions.

How to Build a Remarkable Career in the Food Industry

The food industry is a cornucopia of opportunities, where taste, trends, and innovation merge. From the artistry of culinary creation to the science of food production, it's a field full of flavor and potential. Ready to build a remarkable career in the food industry? Here are the ingredients you need:

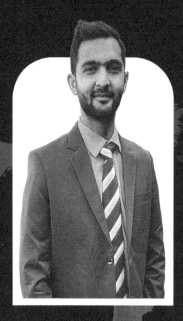

1. Identify Your Area of Interest
Like the courses of a meal, the food industry is multifaceted. You could be a chef , food scientist , nutritionist , restaurant manager , or food marketer . Take some time to explore your interests, skills, and long-term goals to find the right fit.

2. Pursue Relevant Education and Training
Arm yourself with the right tools. This might mean going to culinary school, studying food science, or getting a business degree with a focus on hospitality. Don't forget about apprenticeships and internships, which can offer a taste of real-world experience!

3. Gain Industry Experience
Experience is the best teacher. Seek opportunities in environments that align with your career goals, whether that's a bustling kitchen, a food processing plant, or a corporate food company.

4. Network, Network, Network
Rub elbows with industry insiders. Attend food expos , culinary festivals , and join professional organizations. These connections could lead to exciting opportunities and open doors you never knew existed!

5. Stay Updated and Keep Learning
The food industry is always simmering with new trends and technologies. Stay sharp by attending workshops, webinars, and following industry news. Lifelong learning keeps you ahead of the game.

6. Foster Creativity and Innovation
Creativity is the secret sauce in the food industry. Whether you're crafting new recipes, improving food processing methods, or enhancing dining experiences, thinking outside the box is a valuable skill.

7. Show Commitment and Passion
Love what you do. The food industry can be demanding, but your passion will keep you motivated. Your commitment to creating delicious food and memorable experiences will set you apart.

In the food industry, the recipe for success includes knowing your interests, pursuing education, gaining experience, networking, constant learning, fostering innovation, and showing your passion. Your journey will be as unique as a signature dish, and every step you take will get you closer to a remarkable career in the food industry. Savor the journey and enjoy every bite!

Rajshahi Velvet
Fusion Sauce

Ingredients:

1. 2 cups of tomato sauce
2. 1/2 teaspoon of salt (adjust to taste)
3. 1 to 2 red chillies (adjust for heat), finely chopped
4. 3 tablespoons of butter
5. 3 garlic cloves, minced
6. 1/2 cup of mango chutney (preferably from Rajshahi, if available)
7. 1/4 cup of grated parmesan cheese
8. 1 tablespoon of olive oil (for sautéing)
9. 1/2 to 1 teaspoon smoked paprika (adjust to taste)
10. 1 cup of heavy cream
11. A handful of fresh basil or cilantro leaves, chopped (optional)

Instructions:

1.**Preparation of Ingredients:** Prepare your ingredients by mincing the garlic, chopping the chillies, grating the parmesan, etc.

2.**Sauté Garlic and Chillies:** In a saucepan, heat the olive oil or a tablespoon of butter. Add the minced garlic and chopped red chillies. Sauté until they're fragrant but not browned.

3.**Tomato Sauce and Spices:** Add the tomato sauce and smoked paprika to the pan, mixing well.

4.**Cream Addition:** Pour in the heavy cream and stir. The sauce will start to take on a rich and creamy consistency.

5.**Mango Chutney:** Blend in the mango chutney. This will add a sweet note to balance the heat.

6.**Butter and Parmesan:** On low heat, stir in the butter until it's melted. Add the grated parmesan cheese, stirring until it melts into the sauce.

7.**Seasoning:** Add salt to taste. Adjust the flavor with more smoked paprika or salt as needed.

8.**Herbs:** If you're using basil or cilantro, add them last for a fresh flavor profile.

9.**Serve:** Your Rajshahi Velvet Fusion Sauce is ready! It's great with pasta, as a base for dishes, or drizzled over grilled meats or vegetables.

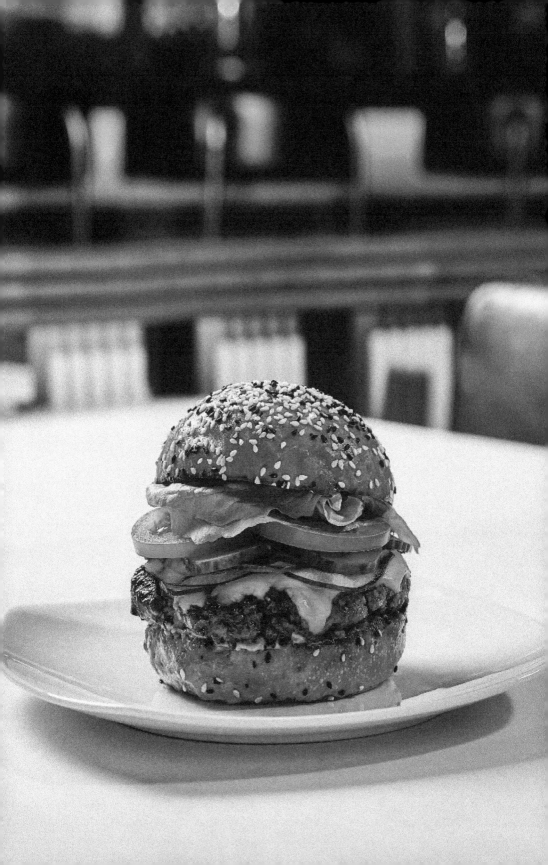

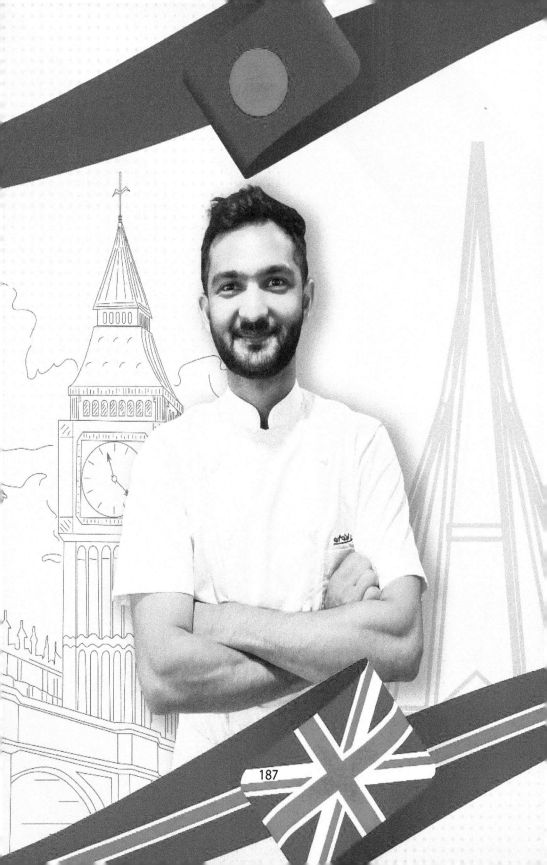

187

Milton Keynes UK
Ingram Content Group UK Ltd.
UKHW052150010224
437043UK00001B/17